W0228143

ACID-BASE REGULATION AND BODY TEMPERATURE

DEVELOPMENTS IN CRITICAL CARE MEDICINE AND ANESTHESIOLOGY

Prakash, O. (ed.): Applied Physiology in Clinical Respiratory Care. 1982. ISBN 90-247-2662-X.

McGeown, Mary G.: Clinical Management of Electrolyte Disorders. 1983. ISBN 0-89838-559-8.

Scheck, P.A., Sjöstrand, U.H., and Smith, R.B. (eds.): Perspectives in High Frequency Ventilation. 1983. ISBN 0-89838-571-7.

Stanley, T.H., and Petty, W.C. (eds.): New Anesthetic Agents, Devices and Monitoring Techniques. 1983. ISBN 0-89838-566-0.

Prakash, O. (ed.): Computing in Anesthesia and Intensive Care. 1983. ISBN 0-89838-602-0.

Stanley, T.H., and Petty, W.C. (eds.): Anesthesia and the Cardiovascular System. 1984. ISBN 0-89838-626-8.

Van Kleef, J.W., Burm, A.G.L., and Spierdijk, J. (eds.): Current Concepts in Regional Anaesthesia. 1984. ISBN 0-89838-644-6.

Prakash, O. (ed.): Critical Care of the Child. 1984. ISBN 0-89838-661-6.

Stanley, T.H., and Petty, W.C. (eds.): Anesthesiology: Today and Tomorrow. 1985. ISBN 0-89838-705-1.

Rahn, H., and Prakash, O. (eds.): Acid-base Regulation and Body Temperature. 1985. ISBN 0-89838-708-6.

ACID-BASE REGULATION AND BODY TEMPERATURE

edited by

HERMANN RAHN, Ph.D.

Department of Physiology
State University of New York at Buffalo
Buffalo, New York
USA

OMAR PRAKASH, M.D.

Thorax Centre and Department of Anesthesia
Erasmus University
Rotterdam
The Netherlands

1985 **MARTINUS NIJHOFF PUBLISHERS**
a member of the KLUWER ACADEMIC PUBLISHERS GROUP
BOSTON / DORDRECHT / LANCASTER

Distributors

for the United States and Canada: Kluwer Academic Publishers, 190 Old Derby
Street, Hingham, MA 02043, USA
for the UK and Ireland: Kluwer Academic Publishers, MTP Press Limited,
Falcon House, Queen Square, Lancaster LA1 1RN, UK
for all other countries: Kluwer Academic Publishers Group, Distribution Center,
P.O. Box 322, 3300 AH Dordrecht, The Netherlands

Library of Congress Cataloging in Publication Data

```
Main entry under title:

Acid-base regulation and body temperature.

    (Developments in critical care medicine and
anesthesiology)
    Includes bibliographies.
    1. Hypothermia, Induced.  2. Acid-base equilibrium.
3. Body temperature--Regulation.  4. Heart--Surgery.
5. Chest--Surgery.  I. Rahn, Hermann, 1912-
II. Prakash, Omar.  III. Series: Developments in
critical care medicine and anaesthesiology.  [DNLM:
1. Acid-Base Equilibrium.  2. Body Temperature.
QU 105 A181]
RD598.A24  1985       612'.01426        85-3070
```

ISBN-13: 978-94-010-8716-2   e-ISBN-13: 978-94-009-5004-7
DOI: 10.1007/978-94-009-5004-7

Copyright

© 1985 by Martinus Nijhoff Publishers, Dordrecht.
Softcover reprint of the hardcover 1st edition 1985
All rights reserved. No part of this publication may be reproduced, stored in a
retrieval system, or transmitted in any form or by any means, mechanical,
photocopying, recording, or otherwise, without the prior written permission of
the publishers,
Martinus Nijhoff Publishers, P.O. Box 163, 3300 AD Dordrecht,
The Netherlands.

Table of contents

Preface

During the last 20 years two groups of investigators have concerned themselves with the problem of acid-base regulation at various body temperatures. Each group, in professional isolation, pursued a separate path. Surgeons and anesthetists developed techniques and tools for hypothermic cardio-pulmonary by-pass operations and based their rationale for acid-base management on in vitro models of blood behavior. Physiologists and biochemists, on the other hand, endeavored to understand acid-base regulation in living organisms naturally subjected to changes in body temperature. Only in the last decade has there been an increasing awareness that each group could benefit from the other's experiences. With this goal in mind members of both groups were invited to present their views and observations in the hope of arriving at a better understanding of acid-base management during hypothermia and gaining a greater insight into the factors which control acid-base regulation during normothermia. This led to the presentation of the present volume with the aim of providing the clinician with a survey of present theories and the resulting strategies for management of the hypothermic patient.

Acknowledgment

The editors express their great appreciation to Miss Augusta Dustan for her dedicated effort in the preparation and editing of the manuscripts.

Contributors

Heinz Becker, M.D.
   Department of Surgery, University of California Medical Center, Los Angeles, Los Angeles, CA 90024, U.S.A.
Gerald D. Buckberg, M.D.
   Department of Surgery, University of California Medical Center, Los Angeles, CA 90024, U.S.A.
Björn Jonson, M.D.
   Department of Clinical Physiology, University of Lund, Lund, Sweden.
Jerry Leaf, M.S.
   Department of Surgery, University of California Medical Center, Los Angeles, Los Angeles, CA 90024, U.S.A.
Andre Malan, Ph.D.
   Laboratoire de Physiologie Respiratoire, Centre National de la Recherche Scientifique, 67087 – Strasbourg, France.
Douglas H. McConnell, M.D.
   Department of Surgery, University of California Medical Center, Los Angeles, Los Angeles, CA 90024, U.S.A.
S.H. Meij, M.S.
   Thorax Centre and the Department of Anesthesia, Erasmus University, Rotterdam, The Netherlands.
Omar Prakash, M.D.
   Thorax Centre and the Department of Anesthesia, Erasmus University, Rotterdam, The Netherlands.
Hermann Rahn, Ph.D.
   Department of Physiology, State University of New York at Buffalo, Buffalo, NY 14214, U.S.A.
R. Blake Reeves, Ph.D.
   Department of Physiology, State University of New York at Buffalo, Buffalo, NY 14214, U.S.A.
John M. Robertson, M.D.
   Department of Surgery, University of California Medical Center, Los Angeles, Los Angeles, CA 90024, U.S.A.

George N. Somero, Ph.D.
Marine Biology Research Division, Scripps Institution of Oceanography, University of California, San Diego, La Jolla, CA 92093, U.S.A.
Henry Swan, M.D.
Professor of Surgery, (Emeritus), University of Colorado School of Medicine, 6700 Lakeridge Road, Lakewood, CO 80227, U.S.A.
Jakob Vinten–Johansen, Ph.D.
Department of Surgery, University of California Medical Center, Los Angeles, Los Angeles, CA 90024, U.S.A.
Fred N. White, Ph.D.
Physiological Research Laboratory, Scripps Institution of Oceanography, University of California, San Diego, La Jolla, CA 92093, U.S.A.

1. Introduction

H. RAHN

During the last three-quarters of this century we have all been imprinted with the truism that normal blood pH is 7.4. We were never told why this particular value was important, and one accepted the fact that somehow this was 'ordained by nature.' Nevertheless, it has served us well, in fact so well that one could easily accept the premise that our respiratory center is a pH-stat responsible for maintaining the appropriate blood reaction. It also led others to conveniently refer to a pH of 7.4 as *neutral* pH and values below or above as acidosis and alkalosis even though, since the times of Claude Bernard, we have known that normal blood is always on the alkaline side of chemical neutrality.

The advent of induced hypothermia in man as a new approach to surgery, some thirty years ago, suddenly placed us in a dilemma, namely, what is the proper acid-base management during body cooling. At that time it was well appreciated that the O_2, CO_2, and pH equilibria were drastically altered when blood was cooled anaerobically, and Severinghaus in 1959 [1] provided us a detailed nomogram describing these changes. For the first time one could predict the simultaneous changes in various blood parameters as blood was cooled. This nomogram might be called an in vitro model of blood behavior, which demonstrated that with body cooling one could no longer maintain the classical relationships of a 37° C acid-base equilibrium.

Because P_{O_2}, P_{CO_2}, and pH were all affected by temperature changes, there were no guidelines, no in vivo models, to tell us which of these, if any, should be kept constant with body cooling. The difficult choice for the anesthesiologist was answered by two different arguments. Severinghaus and Larson in 1965 [2] proposed 'Interaction of decreased metabolism, increased dead space, and increased solubility of CO_2 is such that if ventilation is held constant as body temperature is reduced, arterial P_{CO_2} falls about 40 per cent as temperature falls from 37 to 25° C. It appears desirable to avoid this *low P_{CO_2}* and the *associated alkalosis* from the standpoint of cardiac irritability, so the *addition of CO_2 to inspired gas* has been practiced by some groups doing hypothermic bypass procedures.' (My italics). On the other hand, in 1962 Albers [3], on the basis of another in vitro model, suggested, 'It is concluded that the carbon dioxide content of the arterial blood should be *kept constant* rather than the pH or the carbon dioxide tension.' (My italics).

Thus, one approach suggested that CO_2 be added to the inspired gas in order to keep the pH at normothermic values, while the other approach suggested letting the pH rise and the P_{CO_2} fall in order to maintain the normal value of the blood carbon dioxide content. The former view was generally adopted by most clinical laboratories (see Ream et al.[4] in order to 'avoid this low P_{CO_2} and associated alkalosis' even though it necessitated increasing the P_{CO_2} and the bicarbonate level, while Albers' argument [3] of keeping a normal carbon dioxide content was based on the notion that it would also maintain a constant ratio between hydroxyl and hydrogen ions, a new concept that was ahead of its time.

In the intervening years in vivo models of the behavior of blood during temperature changes were proposed and are discussed in detail in chapters 2, 3, and 4. To quote Williams and Marshall [5] in 1982, these in vivo models 'have opened a new way to investigate this problem. From a biochemical viewpoint there is a strong argument that the appropriate pH and P_{CO_2} are those that give normal values when the blood sample has been anaerobically rewarmed to 37° C. Whether this is also relevant from a physiologic standpoint is not clear, but studies of regional blood flow, oxygen utilization, or neuromuscular function can now be examined with the biochemical set point for a given experimental temperature. On this basis, during hypothermia a low P_{CO_2} and a high pH appear to be reasonable, but further investigation is necessary to show that this biochemical fact is indeed correct physiologically and clinically.'

Introduction to chapters

The first four chapters describe the physiological and biochemical aspects of acid-base regulation, in cold-blooded vertebrates whose body temperature fluctuates with that of the environment, in the peripheral tissues of the shell of warm-blooded animals which are cooler than that of their core, and in hibernating mammals. The last three chapters are concerned with a discussion of these in vivo models and other strategies as they relate to acid-base management of hypothermic patients.

In Chapter 2 Reeves shows first of all that in man the so-called normal acid-base values of a pH of 7.4 and a P_{CO_2} of 40 torr exist only in the core thermostated at 37° C, while in the shell our cooler peripheral tissues are continuously exposed to higher pH and lower P_{CO_2} values. The opposite holds true for tissues warmer than the core, such as the liver and exercising muscles. In these tissues pH and P_{CO_2} will deviate markedly from those of the core but the Donnan ratio, the plasma bicarbonate concentration, and the hydroxyl/hydrogen ion ratio remain unaltered. The reason for this behavior resides in the ubiquitous presence in blood and tissues of the protein, imidazole of histidine, whose pK changes with temperature in such a manner that the protein net charge remains constant. The constant dissociation of this compound is expressed as an alpha value, hence alpha-stat regulation, in contrast to pH-stat regulation. Alpha-stat regulation not only occurs in warm-blooded animals whose tissues are warmer and colder than the core, but also in air-breathing ectotherms (cold-blooded vertebrates) as their daily body temperature changes.

Malan, in Chapter 3, discusses the acid-base strategy of hibernating mammals. When the body cools, the blood does not follow alpha-stat regulation but maintains nearly normothermic pH and P_{CO_2} values. This is accomplished by a profound reduction in ventilation, retention of CO_2, a large increase in bicarbonate concentration, and can be likened to a compensated respiratory acidosis. While their blood behavior provides an excellent example of pH-stat regulation, it is important to point out that recent findings indicate that certain vital tissues, such as the heart and liver, follow alpha-stat regulation.

The enzymatic consequences under alpha-stat regulation are described in Chapter 4. Somero and White discuss the importance of conserving the fractional protonation state, or alpha-stat regulation, for enzymes like lactate dehydrogenase, and other enzymes such as phosphofructokinase (PFK) having histidyl residues, in order to conserve binding ability and catalytic reserve capacity at various temperatures. As long as the change in intracellular pH with temperature follows the same change as the pK of imidazole of histidine, alpha-stat regulation is maintained and conserves the structural and functional properties of enzymes and other proteins. On the other hand, during hibernation with pH-stat regulation of the blood, the PFK activity will be completely abolished and muscle glycolysis (necessary later for locomotor activity and body warming following arousal) fully inhibited. While intracellular muscle pH of the hibernator follows pH-stat strategy of the blood, the intracellular pH of the heart and liver follows alpha-stat regulation, suggesting that for these vital tissues specialized regulatory mechanisms are available for proton extrusion which preserves their normal net protein charge.

With these in vivo models of acid-base regulation as a background, we now turn to the clinical management of patients subjected to hypothermia for various surgical interventions. In Chapter 5 Swan discusses four fundamental strategies for acid-base management during hypothermic cardiopulmonary by-pass operations, including alpha-stat and pH-stat strategies. These are illustrated on a pH-P_{CO_2}-temperature diagram and also demonstrate clearly why the reporting of 'temperature corrected' blood values is undesirable. Of particular interest is Swan's historical review of various clinical practices of acid-base management in the past and how they pass muster today.

The application of alpha-stat strategy during hypothermia in infants is described in Chapter 6 by Prakash, Jonson, and Meij. This is achieved by maintaining normothermic ventilation as the infant is cooled and monitoring continuously the expired gas for CO_2. The technique for CO_2 monitoring is described in detail and its usefulness emphasized because in infants blood monitoring may be limited. A brief review is provided of other clinics which have employed alpha-stat strategy in adult patients.

The last chapter, 7, by Buckberg and associates, deals with an experimental model of acid-base regulation in dogs subjected to hypothermia. The objectives were to measure the blood flow to various organs, particularly the heart, interrupt the flow, and compare the recovery when animals had been subjected to profound alkalosis while control animals were subjected to alpha-stat regulation. While alpha-stat regulation may be ideal for organ systems which are continuously perfused, their results show that after interruption of blood flow, the recovery of animals subjected to the alkaline strategy was superior to those maintained by alpha-stat management.

A simplified overview of acid-base regulation is shown below in Fig. 1, where the arrows indicate three general strategies of acid-base regulation as body temperature is reduced from 37°C. The middle arrow represents the in vivo alpha-stat strategy representing the peripheral tissues of warm-blooded animals which are cooler than their core temperature. It also represents the blood behavior of ectotherms as their daily body temperature fluctuates with that of their environment.

The lower arrow represents the in vivo strategy found in the blood of mammalian hibernators, a constant pH strategy. It reflects a compensated respiratory acidosis and is similar to the strategy presently employed in most clinical settings.

The top arrow respresents a region of induced respiratory alkalosis. No in vivo model for this strategy is known and it is based on experimental results presented by Buckberg, demonstrating that cardiac function is greatly improved over constant alpha or constant pH strategy.

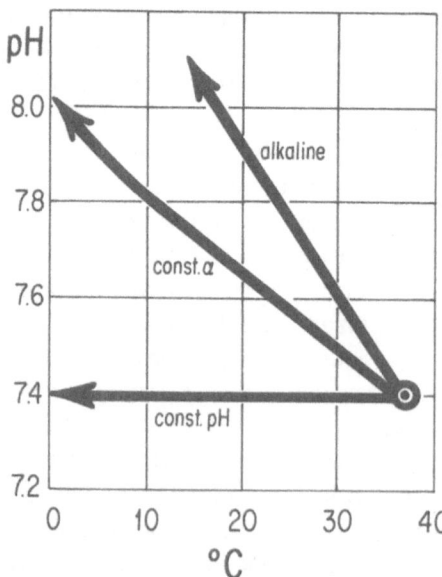

Fig. 1. Starting at a pH = 7.4 at 37°C, these arrows describe three acid-base strategies as described in text.

Retrospect

The first description of the alpha-stat model of acid-base regulation by Reeves in 1972 [6] was an attempt to explain earlier observations that ectotherms at various body temperatures regulate their blood to maintain a constant ratio of hydroxyl to hydrogen ions, (OH^-/H^+), rather than to preserve a constant pH (Fig. 2). At that time the regulation of a constant OH^-/H^+ ratio appeared to provide a new way of looking at acid-base regulation [7]. It is embarrassing to admit that even ten years ago we were unaware that similar concepts had emerged previously and independently in several laboratories to explain acid-base regulation, particularly when body temperature was altered. In 1978 we made our amends [8], reviewing various studies that had been previously ignored and forgotten by us as well as others, starting with the reflections of Benjamin Moore, Professor of Biochemistry at Oxford. These were published in an abstract in the Proceedings of the

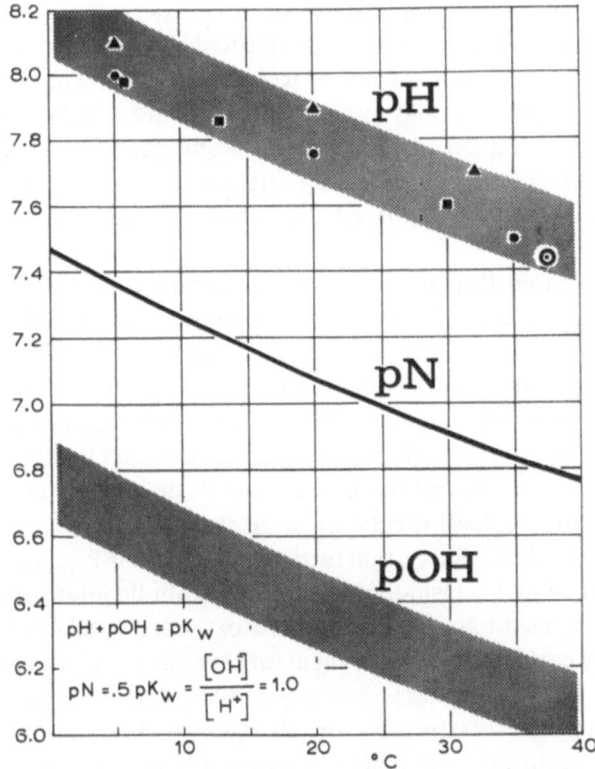

Fig. 2. Arterial blood pH values of various unanesthetized ectotherms living at various body temperatures. These values parallel the chemical neutrality of water, pN, derived from the table of physical constants shown in Fig. 3. The lower shaded area represents the pOH of arterial blood (see text). From Rahn 1967 [7].

Physiological Society, October 1919 [9]. While not specifically concerned with changes in temperature, it is possibly the earliest reference to an OH^-/H^+ ratio.

The cause of the exquisite sensitivity of living cells to changes in hydrogen- and hydroxyl-ion concentration. By Benjamin Moore.

'It is now universally accepted that changes in hydrogen-ion and hydroxyl-ion concentration which lie almost within the limits of detection produce a profound effect upon living organisms. Life is only possible within short range of the neutral point.

This has puzzled me for many years and it is only recently that the meaning of it has dawned upon me.

The large number of workers who have worked upon the subject may be divided into two groups, namely, those who express their results in terms of hydrogen-ion concentration and those who express them in terms of hydroxyl-ion concentration. It is this conventional method of expression which has obscured the truth, for the effects of changes in concentration of the two ions upon an amphoteric system are proportional not to the concentration of either ion but to the ratio of the concentrations of the two ions'.

Much credit for his insight must be given to J.H. Austin, a student of Van Slyke, who in 1922 became Professor of Research Medicine at the University of Pennsylvania. In 1925 [10] and 1927 [11] he and his collaborators presented experimental results and an elegant analysis, leading them to advocate what we today would call regulation of a constant OH^-/H^+ ratio when body temperature of a cold-blooded vertebrate is altered. These studies seemed to have been totally ignored.

In 1954 Winterstein [12], unaware of Austin and Cullin's contribution, developed a similar concept. Using the Winterstein concept, Albers in 1962 [3] developed a blood nomogram for the calculation of the OH^-/H^+ ratio as a function of temperature and advocated that during hypothermia in man one should allow the pH to go up and the P_{CO_2} to fall in order to maintain the normal carbon dioxide content of the blood as well as the normal OH^-/H^+ ratio, a rather prophetic statement in view of the in vivo models developed later.

Our interests in acid-base regulation were stimulated by the observations of Robin [13] in 1962, who reported that turtles changed their P_{CO_2} and pH with body temperature but in such a fashion that they could not be interpreted by classical concepts of $37°C$ acid-base regulation. We extended similar studies to other species and were careful to acclimate them for several days to a given temperature before arterial blood samples were drawn. Only later we learned that such precautions were unnecessary, since the changes we observed were not acclimations at all but occurred immediately with cooling in a manner similar to that observed when anaerobic blood samples are cooled or warmed, namely, shifts in physico-chemical equilibria. It is also important to note that all our blood samples were drawn from unanesthetized animals with implanted catheters and that the pH and P_{CO_2} measurements were made at the body temperature of the animals.

7

These observations showed that as body temperature fell arterial pH increased and P_{CO_2} fell in a rather precise fashion [7], and over the years subsequent experiments revealed the same pattern in all the ectothermic air breathers [14, 15, 16, 17]. Fig. 2 shows the arterial blood pH of frogs, toads, and turtles at various body temperatures. At first this behavior was rather puzzling until we realized that the changes in pH paralleled the pH changes in chemically neutral water, which we have labeled pN.

Chemical neutrality. At that time little attention had been paid to the biological implications of the large changes in the dissociation constant of water, pKw, as a function of temperature. As water cools it dissociates less, as shown on the right hand ordinate of Fig. 3. Its dissociation into OH^- and H^+ ions allows one to calculate the pH of chemical neutrality, pN, at any temperature, which is equal to 0.5 pKw. This is shown on the left ordinate of Fig. 2, where pN changes from 6.8 at 37.5° C to 7.4 at 3° C.

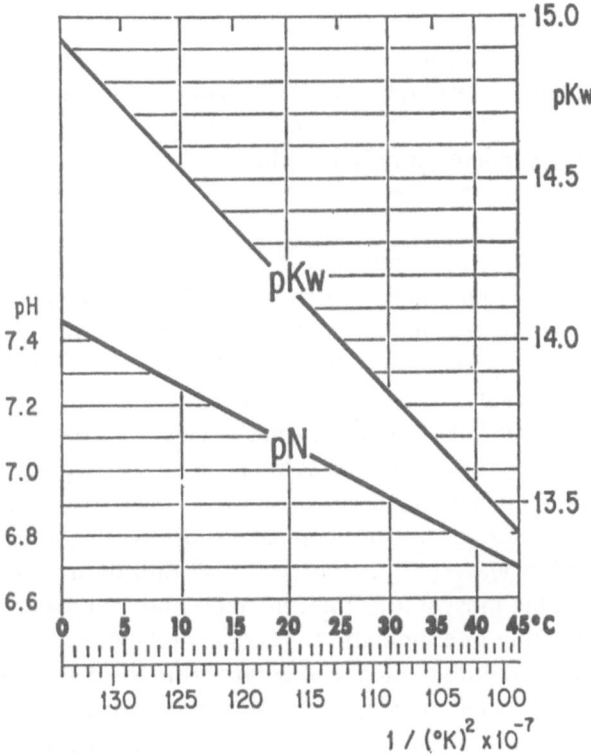

Fig. 3. Changes in pKw and pN = (0.5 pKw) with temperature. Plotted from Handbook of Chemistry and Physics (1956).

Concept of a constant relative alkalinity. The parallelism between the blood pH and neutral pH of water in Fig. 2 is striking and reflects the regulation of *constant relative alkalinity,* i.e., an alkalinity relative to the chemical neutrality of water (Howell *et al.* [14]). This behavior over a large temperature range confirms the classical observations of Peters and Van Slyke [18], whose opening sentence in their chapter on acid-base balance states, 'During more than half a century it has been recognized that for the maintenance in the organism of a state compatible with life the reactions of the inner fluids must be slightly to the alkaline side of the neutral point, and that much deviation from this physiological reaction is disastrous.'

Concept of a constant (OH^-/H^+) ratio. The constant relative alkalinity can also be described quantitatively in terms of a *constant OH^-/H^+ ratio.* If the blood pH is known, one can also calculate the blood pOH, since at any temperature pH + pOH = pKw. The changes in pOH are shown in Fig. 2 and also parallel the line of neutrality, pN. The difference, (pH − pOH), = (log H^+ − log OH^-) = ca. 1.4 units in Fig. 2. The antilog of 1.4, or 25, describes the constant ratio of 25 OH^- ions for every H^+ ion, (OH^-/H^+ = 25), which is maintained in these animals over the whole temperature range. Note also in Fig. 2 the blood pH of 7.4 for man at 37.5°C. The ionization constant of water, pKw, at this temperature (Fig. 3) is 13.6, and therefore his blood pOH = (13.6 − 7.4) or 6.2. Since the (pH − pOH) = 1.2, the regulated OH^-/H^+ ratio of man is 16:1, the antilog of 1.2. Chemical neutrality, pN, at this temperature is 6.8, which is close to the intracellular pH of his tissues.

Intracellular pH. The first measurements of intracellular pH in various tissues as a function of body temperature in ectotherms were done by Malan *et al.* [19]. With the exception of heart muscle, all showed a $\Delta pH/\Delta T$ slope similar to that observed in the blood. Furthermore, the tissue pH values were all close to pN, the line of chemical neutrality. Thus one can further generalize by describing the OH^-/H^+ ratio of intracellular compartments of close to 1.0 and the difference between the extra- and intracellular pH as a constant over the temperature range. These are discussed in Chapter 2.

A possible explanation for the intracellular pH of tissue near the neutrality of water was provided by Davis [20]. He surveyed the ionization constant of several hundred water-soluble biosynthetic intermediates and found with a few exceptions that these fleeting intermediaries are completely ionized in the region of neutrality and thus had little tendency to escape from the cell across the plasma membrane. He argued that complete ionization is an efficient retention mechanism for metabolites within the cell or organelle, a concept that was elegantly expressed in the title of his paper, 'On the Importance of Being Ionized.'

Arterial P_{CO_2} and ventilation. As the in vivo pH increases with fall in body temperature, the arterial P_{CO_2} decreases rapidly without, however, changing the plasma bicarbonate concentration or the CO_2 stores of the blood and tissues [6]. The P_{CO_2} is determined by the ratio of CO_2 production to ventilation. As temperature falls, CO_2 production falls, but ventilation in these animals changes relatively little, if at all [21], accounting for the fall in arterial P_{CO_2}. One may, therefore postulate that a constant OH^-/H^+ ratio is achieved by the response of the respiratory center which regulates ventilation to metabolic CO_2 production in such a manner that at every temperature the P_{CO_2} is adjusted to the changes in the CO_2 solubility and pK' of CO_2 dissociation, leaving the plasma bicarbonate concentration and the CO_2 stores of the tissues unaltered. This control of the respiratory center in man and lower vertebrates will be discussed in Chapter 2.

The alpha-stat concept. As ectotherms cool or warm, certain blood and tissue properties are kept constant, and presumably regulated, while pH and P_{CO_2} are greatly altered. Obviously, these animals do not have a pH-stat in the classical sense. The CO_2 stores of the tissues and the plasma bicarbonate level are maintained. Thus, in spite of large changes in P_{CO_2} these animals are not concerned with loading or unloading their CO_2 stores. Furthermore, the OH^-/H^+ ratio of ca. 25:1 in their blood is maintained, while their tissue pH is near chemical neutrality. Lastly, the intracellular/extracellular ratio of electrolytes, the Donnan ratio, is preserved. The question remains, what are the advantages of this regulation and what are the responsible buffer systems?

The observation described in Fig. 2 led Albery and Lloyd [22] to suggest that a buffer system which would support this behavior would have to have a pK of approximately 7.0 and a ΔH of approximately 7 kcal $\cdot$ mol^{-1}. Phosphate and bicarbonate buffers do not answer this description. Reeves [16], however, showed that the peptide imidazole of histidine, available in decimolar concentrations in our blood and tissues, does answer this prediction with its pK of 6.9 at 25° C and a ΔH of 6.9 kcal $\cdot$ mol^{-1}. The change in pK of histidyl imidazole with temperature is essentially the same as the change in neutrality of water. Thus the slopes with temperature of pK of histidyl imidazole, pN, pHi, and pH blood are similar and any given OH$^-$/H$^+$ ratio describes a finite degree of dissociation, or alpha value of imidazole of histidine (Chapter 2, Fig. 10). Alpha-stat regulation provides a constant protein net charge, an important enviroment for preserving the structural and functional properties and optimal reaction rates of temperature-sensitive enzyme systems and other proteins. These are described by Somero and White in Chapter 4.

Since many of the considerations in this book are based on the interpretation of in vivo models, I have listed below in alphabetical order various reviews of in vivo acid-base regulations that have appeared during the last few years.

10

General reviews of in vivo models

Cohen JJ, Kassirer JP: Comparative acid-base physiology. In: Acid/Base, Little Brown, Boston, Cohen JJ, Kassirer JP (eds). 1982: 465–480.

Jackson DC: Strategies of blood acid-base control in ectothermic vertebrates. In: A Companion to Animal Physiology, Taylor CR, Johansen K, Bolis L (eds). Cambridge University Press, Cambridge, 1982: 73–90.

Malan A. Respiration and acid-base state in hibernation. In: Hibernation and Torpor in Mammals and Birds, Lyman CP, Willis JS, Malan A, Wang LCH (eds). Academic Press, New York, 1982: 237–282.

Rahn H, Reeves BR, Howell BJ: Hydrogen ion regulation, temperature and evolution. Am Rev Respir Dis 112: 165–172, 1975.

Rahn H, Reeves RB, Hydrogen ion regulation during hypothermia: from the Amazon to the Operating Room. In: Applied Physiology in Clinical Respiratory Care, Prakash O (ed). Martinus Nijhoff Publ., The Hague, 1982: 1–15.

Reeves RB: The interaction of body temperature and acid-base balance in ectothermic vertebrates. Ann Rev Physiol 39: 559–586, 1977.

Reeves RB, Rahn H: Patterns in vertebrate acid-base regulation. In: Evolution of Respiratory Processes: A Comparative Approach, Wood S, Lenfant C (eds). Marcel Dekker, New York, 1979: 225–252.

Swan H: The hydroxyl-hydrogen ion concentration ratio during hypothermia. Surg Gynecol Obstet 155: 897–912, 1982.

Truchot JP: L'equilibre acido-basique extracellulaire et sa regulation dans les divers groupes animaux. J Physiol Paris 77: 529–580, 1981.

White FN: A comparative physiological approach to hypothermia – Editorial. J Thorac Cardiovasc Surg 82: 821–831, 1981.

White FN, Somero G: Acid-base regulation and phospholipid adaptation to temperature: time courses and physiological significance of modifying the milieu for protein function. Physiol Rev 62: 40–90, 1982.

References

1. Severinghaus JW: Respiration and hypothermia. Ann New York Acad Sci 80: 384–394, 1959.
2. Severinghaus JW, Larson EP Jr: Respiration in Anesthesia. In: Handbook of Respiration, Vol. 2, Fenn WO, Rahn H (eds). Am Physiol Soc Washington, 1965: 1219–1257.
3. Albers C: Die ventilatorische Kontrolle der Saüre-Basen-Gleichgewicht in Hypothermie. Anaesthesist 11: 43–51, 1962.
4. Ream AK, Reitz BA, Silverberg G: Temperature correction of P_{CO_2} and pH in estimating acid-base status. Anesthesiol 56: 41–44, 1982.
5. Williams JJ, Marshall BE: A fresh look at an old question. Anesthesiol 56: 1–2, 1982.
6. Reeves RB: An imidazole alphastat hypothesis for vertebrate acid–base regulation. Respir Physiol 14: 219–236, 1972.
7. Rahn H: Gas transport from the external environment to the cell. In: Development of the Lung, deReuck AVS, Porter R. (eds). Ciba Foundation Symposium. J and A Churchill, London, 1967: 3–23.

8. Rahn H, Howell BJ: The OH^-/H^+ concept of acid-base balance: Historical development. Respir Physiol 33: 91–97, 1978.

9. Moore B: The cause of the exquisite sensitivity of living cells to changes in hydrogen and hydroxyl-ion concentration. J Physiol (London) 53:LVII–LVIII, 1919.

10. Austin JH, Cullen GE: Hydrogen ion concentration of the blood in health and disease. Medicine 4: 275–343, 1925.

11. Austin JH, Sunderman FW, Camack JG: Studies in serum electrolytes. II. The electrolyte composition and the pH of serum of a poikilothermous animal at different temperatures. J Biol Chem 72: 677–685, 1927.

12. Winterstein H: Der Einfluss der Körpertemperatur auf das Saüre-Basen-Gleichgewicht in Blut. Naunyn–Schmiedebergs Arch Exp Pathol Pharmakol 223: 1–18, 1954.

13. Robin ED: Relationship between temperature and plasma pH and carbon dioxide tension in the turtle. Nature (London) 195: 249–251, 1962.

14. Howell BJ, Baumgardner FW, Bondi K, Rahn H: Acid-base balance in cold-blooded vertebrates as a function of body temperature. Am J Physiol 218: 600–606, 1970.

15. Howell BJ, Rahn H: Regulation of acid-base balance in reptiles. In: Biology of the Reptilia, Vol. 5, Gans C, Dawson WR (eds). Academic Press, London, 1976: 335–363.

16. Reeves RB: The interaction of body temperature and acid-base balance in ectothermic vertebrates. Ann Rev Physiol 39: 559–586, 1977.

17. Reeves RB, Rahn H: Patterns in vertebrate acid-base regulation. In: Evolution of respiratory processes: A Comparative Approach, Wood S, Lenfant C (eds). Marcel Dekker, New York, 1979: 225–252.

18. Peters JP, Van Slyke DD: Quantitative Clinical Chemistry. Williams and Wilkins, Baltimore, 1932: 868.

19. Malan A, Wilson TL, Reeves RB: Intracellular pH in cold-blooded vertebrates as a function of body temperature. Respir Physiol 28: 29–47, 1976.

20. Davis BD: On the importance of being ionized. Arch Biochem Biophys 78: 497–509, 1958.

21. Jackson DC: Strategies of blood acid-base control in ectothermic vertebrates. In: A Companion to Animal Physiology, Taylor CR, Johansen K, Bolis L (eds). Cambridge University Press, Cambridge, 1982: 73–90.

22. Albery WJ, Lloyd BB: Variation of chemical potential with temperature. In: Development of the Lung, deReuck AVS, Porter R (eds). J and A Churchill Ltd, London, 1967: 30–33.

2. What are normal acid-base conditions in man when body temperature changes?

ROBERT BLAKE REEVES

Introduction

Over the short time span of 25 years the use of general body hypothermia for cardiac surgery has progressed from experimental to commonplace. In 1983 the total number of patients on whom hypothermia was employed in the United States alone exceeded 170,000. Moreover, it is now accepted that induction of and recovery from hypothermia carries minimal risks. The widespread practice of whole body hypothermia has raised the practical question of what constitutes correct acid-base management during hypothermia. This question had previously been ignored because, although principles of acid-base regulation at 37° C are well known, extension of basic theory to other body temperatures appeared of no particular utility.

The human body even when registering a nomal core temperature, is not,how ever, an isothermal system. Acid-base investigations had long ignored the well-established fact that large regional differences from core temperature exist in man. Thus there must always be tissues operating normally in a regulated acid-base environment that are significantly displaced in temperature from core. What then is the normal acid-base state of peripheral tissues when operating temperatures at these sites exceeds or falls below core temperature? The answer appears to be not a state of constant pH as temperature changes, but rather a state whereby protein ionization is protected from variation. This chapter reviews recent evidence on this point and demonstrates that the answer is, in a phylogenetic sense, an ancient one that man shares with most vertebrates, warm- or cold-blooded. The serendipitous benefits of this inquiry go well beyond the practical utility of an acid-base management schema for hypothermia. A dividend of incorporating temperature in the analysis of acid-base problems is to view the whole process of acid-base regulaion from a new broader perspective. This analysis offers as a bonus answer to the questions of why is acid-base regulation necessary (i.e. what is being regulated?) and the related question of why pH 7.40 at 37° C?

Regional temperature inhomogeneity in normal man

The classical principles of acid-base analysis apply to an isothermal system at 37 degrees; the normal human body is, however, not uniformly isothermal for in most human activities localized tissue temperatures may depart significantly from regulated core temperature. Figure 1 provides an example of how such regional temperature differences can be maintained with a normothermic core. This illustration derives from the classical studies of intravascular temperatures first made with thermocouple-catheters by Bazett et al.[1]. If the hand is kept immersed in a cold bath, the arterial blood in the limb is cooled by venous blood returning from the cold distal tissues. Thus blood leaves the normothermic heart and lungs with normal acid-base values and is cooled transit in the arterial vessels. The change in blood temperature occurs without change in gas content, in particular, without change in carbon dioxide content. Only when blood reaches the arteriolar-capillary vessels does gas exchange occur, discharging oxygen and loading carbon dioxide. Venous blood returning to the heart after gas exchange takes place is warmed again by a process of heat exchange at constant gas content.

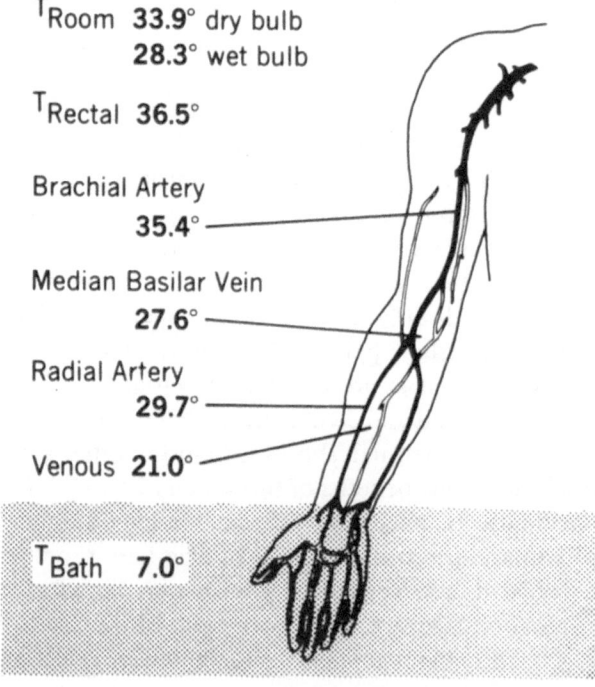

TRoom **33.9°** dry bulb
28.3° wet bulb

TRectal **36.5°**

Brachial Artery
35.4°

Median Basilar Vein
27.6°

Radial Artery
29.7°

Venous **21.0°**

TBath **7.0°**

Fig. 1. Cooling of arterial blood in transit in the arteries as a result of rewarming of cold blood returning in adjacent veins from a cold water immersed hand. (After Bazett et al.[1]).

Acid-base consequences of variable temperature

The effect of temperature change on blood pH and CO_2 partial pressure can be measured accurately for these conditions in vitro. Measured values for normal human blood under these conditions are shown in Fig. 2. The response to cooling is a significant increase in blood pH. The rate of pH change with temperature is about $-.015$ units/$^\circ$C; more precisely, the pH-temperature coefficient increases as temperature falls [2]. The simultaneous variation of carbon dioxide tension with blood temperature change is also shown in Fig. 2; CO_2 tension falls non-linearly as temperature decreases. In the superficial capillaries of the hand at 7° C, the pH and P_{CO_2} of the blood *before gas exchange* are 7.84 and 8 torr, respectively. Analogous blood measurement have been made for a wide variety of conditions; the observed temperature coefficients are remarkably insensitive to initial acid-base conditions and to moderate variations in hematocrit [2].

Normal blood acid-base status, as found in the microcirculation of tissues operating over a range of temperatures around core, encompasses a wide range of values for pH and P_{CO_2}. Figure 3 illustrates the extensive variety of normal acid-base states demonstrable under conditions reflecting normal human activity. The pH of blood leaving the heart with a value of 7.40 at 37° is increased or decreased depending upon whether the blood, in transit at constant CO_2 content, is cooled or warmed. Blood perfusing tissues in a cold hand at 20° has a pH of 7.66 and a P_{CO_2} of 16 torr, while comparable blood acid-base conditions for maximally working muscle with a temperature of 42° are found to be 7.35 and 47 torr. Once gas exchange occurs, blood from these sites will return to a common core temperature, again changing pH and P_{CO_2} values en route, with typical mixed venous values of 7.36 and 47 torr. Clearly, each tissue temperature dictates a different normal acid-base state in terms of pH and P_{CO_2} values. The salient feature of this analysis is recognition of the fact that *normal* acid-base status

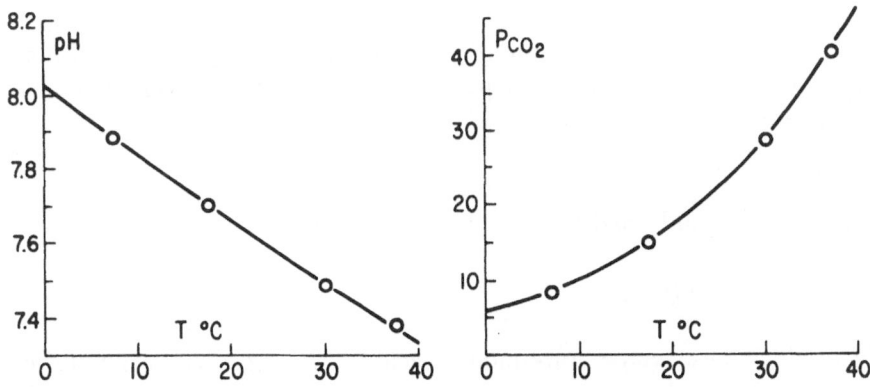

Fig. 2. Changes in pH and partial pressure in torr of carbon dioxide (P_{CO_2}) of human whole blood when temperature is altered at constant normal CO_2 content (after Reeves [2]).

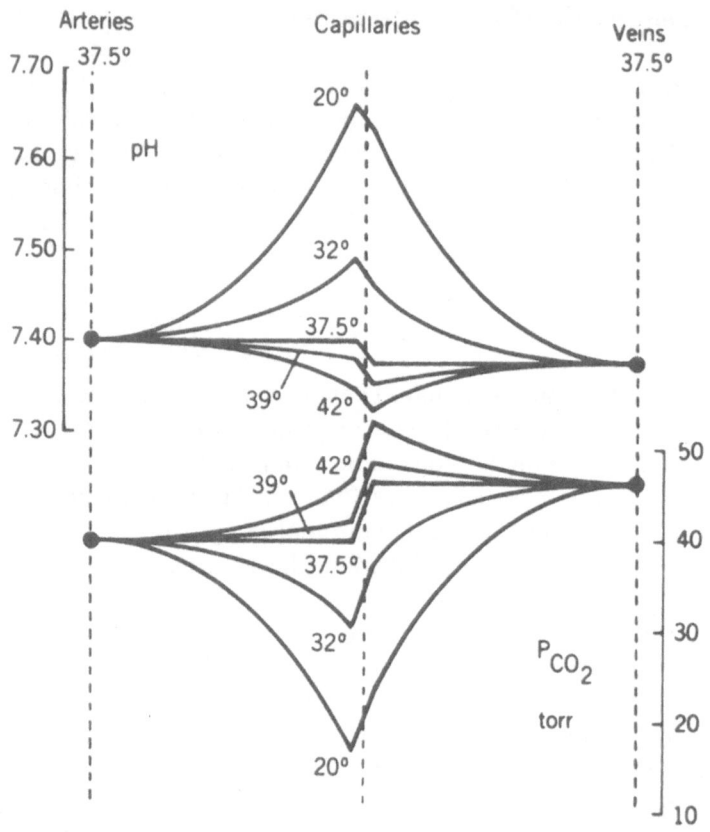

Fig. 3. Schematic diagram depicting the effect on blood pH and P_{CO_2} of normothermic blood perfusing vascular beds at temperatures different from core temperature. These values are computed for arterial blood of pH 7.40 and P_{CO_2} of 40 Torr (37.5°C) containing .025 mol/l plasma carbon dioxide content. Temperatures illustrated are typical of the following: cold skin, 20°C; cold skeletal muscle, 32°C; coronary bed, 37.5°C; liver, 39°C; exercising muscle, 42°C. After Reeves [2].

requires a different set of pH and P_{CO_2} values *at each temperature* and that the magnitude of these temperature dependent changes from normothermic values is indeed large.

Origin of observed behavior

Role of protein buffers

The origin of these temperature-induced acid-base changes has been fully delineated [2, 3]. These phenomena are quantitatively predicted from the binary buffer properties of whole blood; these principles also apply to intracellular fluids. Whole blood and intracellular fluid constitute a mixture of CO_2-bicarbonate and protein buffers. Acting under conditions where exchange of CO_2 is ruled out, the buffer value of the CO_2bicarbonate conjugate acid-base pair is only from 12 to 20% of the buffer value attributable to protein. Hence protein is the predominant buffer both in whole blood and cytoplasm and the effect of temperature on protein buffering largely determines the response of pH and P_{CO_2}.

Protein histidyl imidazole groups: principal physological buffer

Of the 20 genetically coded amino acids constituting all proteins, one, Histidine, is the focus of acid-base regulation; the key role of this amino acid in acid-base balance is only made apparent when temperature change enters the picture. Amino acids in amide linkage comprise the primary polypeptide structure of proteins; these amino acids have side chains that attach to the alpha carbon. Four amino acids have hydrophobic R-group side chains which cause them to remain buried within a globular protein molecule away from the aqueous environment of cytoplasm or plasma. Seven amino acids, including histidine, have side chains that are so polar, or hydrophilic, that they prefer the aqueous environment on the outside of a protein. The remaining amino acids are ambivalent in being neither so polar they must be in the aqueous phase nor so hydrophobic they must remain inside the protein molecule.

A hallmark of the hydrophilic amino acids is their propensity to bear a charge. Aspartic and glutamic acids have carboxyl groups which, at physiological pH values, lose a proton, giving their side chains a negative charge. Amide derivatives of these amino acids, asparagine and glutamine, have no negative charge, but are so polar they, too, remain on the surface of the protein. Lysine and arginine have nitrogen atoms with unused electron pairs that attract protons at physiological pH values, imparting to these side chain groups a positive charge. Histidine's side chain imidazole ring also has unpaired electrons that can bind a proton and thus cause the imidazole ring to bear a positive charge (Fig. 4). However, the affinity of histidine's imidazole ring for protons is relatively weak such that in vivo roughly only half the imidazole rings bear a positive charge, and the remainder are uncharged.

Only histidine's imidazole R-group binds a proton reversibly over the physiological pH range of 6–8. Hence it is this group, well-represented in all proteins, that is the principal buffer of the cell. Because the act of binding a proton converts an uncharged histidine imidazole side chain into a positively charged group, proton binding not only alters the net protein charge, but it also alters charge-charge interactions on the surface of the protein. Interactions between charges on the surface of the protein importantly affect the conformation of the protein and the association of sub-units. Moreover, histidine imidazoles also play a key role at the active site of many enzymes where their protonation state directly affects activity. Hence supplying a protein with protons simultaneously (1) promotes

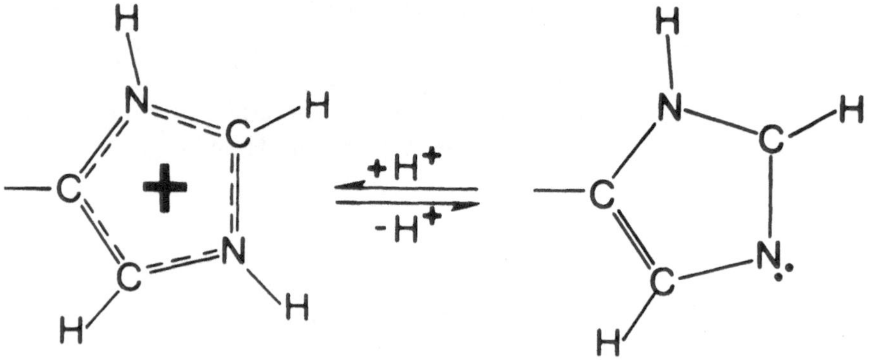

Fig. 4. The histidyl imidazole R-group showing the change in imidazole ring charge state when protonated. Notation used in text for proton binding equilibrium of histidyl imidazole (Im) ring is also shown.

proton binding or buffering, (2) alters the net charge on the protein, (3) affects the conformation of the protein, and (4) alters enzymatic function. All protein functions, like enzymatic activity, or the binding of small molecular weight substrates and allosteric modulators, are exquisitely sensitive to these alterations in histidine imidazole charge state. Thus control of protein function via adjustment of the fraction of histidine imidazole groups bearing a proton is the central objective of acid-base regulation. In blood and extra-cellular fluid, the balance between protonated and unprotonated histidine imidazole groups is achieved by controlling the plasma pH via combined ventilatory control of carbon dioxide tension and renal control of strong ion (buffer base) concentration. Intracellularly, active control of strong ion concentrations by ion transport pumps in the plasma membrane determines intracellular pH and thus regulates cytoplasmic peptide histidine imidazole charge state.

The pK of the histidyl imidazole group lies directly in the middle of the physiological pH range 6–8; we shall argue later the inverse of this statement better describes the situation in vivo: viz., the physiological pH range has, through selection, come to correspond to the range of pK_{Im} values in proteins. One must explicitly recognize, however, that all histidine imidazoles do not possess the same pK_{Im}. Much functional importance attaches in specific situations for biasing the ionization state of a particular imidazole group to serve a particular reaction mechanism requirement. Because of electrostatic interactions within proteins the range of microscopic pK values for protein histidine imidazole groups can be large. For instance in a typical well-studied globular protein, deoxyhemoglobin A, eleven specific alpha and beta chain microscopic histidine pK_{Im} values have been independently measured with [13] C NMR; they average 7.12 with a range of 6.25 to 8.2 [4]. In addition to histidine imidazole, N-terminal amino groups also contribute to protein buffering, but their lesser concentration limits their contribution to total protein buffering to less than 10%. Again using data from hemoglobin [4], the range of microscopic pK values for alpha amino ionizations is from 6.9 to 7.8, indistinguishable from that of histidine imidazole groups. For the sake of clarity of exposition, all physiological protein buffer groups will be collectively referred to as simply histidine-imidazole. The proton equilibrium for histidine imidazole can be written as shown in Fig. 4

$$HIm^+ = H^+ + Im$$

and the fraction of the total histidine imidazoles in the un-protonated form can be calculated as

$$\alpha = [Im] / ([HIm^+] + [Im]) = b / (1 + b)$$

where $b = 10^{(pH - pK_{Im})}$ and pK_{Im} is the negative logarithm of the equilibrium constant for the imidazole proton dissociation reaction. Note that when the difference $(pH - pK_{Im})$ remains constant, α is constant.

From the viewpoint of temperature change the parameter of central interest is the enthalpy of dissociation of histidine imidazole groups, a measure of the change in pK_{Im} with temperature. Measurements obtained for histidine residues in stripped hemoglobin as well as a mixture of plasma proteins, each in the absence of small molecular buffer species like phosphates, yield a value for $\Delta H° = 7 \, kcal/mol$ [2]. This necessarily is a global value reflecting the average behavior of individual histidine imidazole groups whose individual microscopic enthalpies in intact proteins can be fully as variable as their respective pK_{Im} values. The net effect is shown in Fig. 5; the average dpK_{Im}/dT is about $-.019$ units/°C. This is a strong dependence of pK_{Im} on temperature, much greater than the corresponding change in pK' for CO_2-bicarbonate (-0.002 to -0.011 units/°C, at 37° and 7°C, respectively). The fact that both protein histidine imidazole buffering and pK temperature coefficient predominate over those of carbonic acid signifies that when temperature varies at constant CO_2 content, the properties of the protein buffer groups principally determine the behavior of the total system (blood or tissue) pH and P_{CO_2} response.

Interaction between CO_2 and protein histidyl imidazole groups

In order to embrace the complexity of acid-base regulation in vivo, it is helpful to review the interaction of carbonic acid and protein histidine imidazole groups, the two components of the binary buffer system of blood, first at constant temperature. Figure 6 shows the titration of whole blood with carbon dioxide at 37°. The lower panel depicts the CO_2 combining curve showing total carbon dioxide as a function of CO_2 partial pressure. The total CO_2 is the sum of bicarbonate ion and dissolved CO_2 concentrations; the latter amounts to only about 5% of the total and is a linear function of partial pressure. The increase in

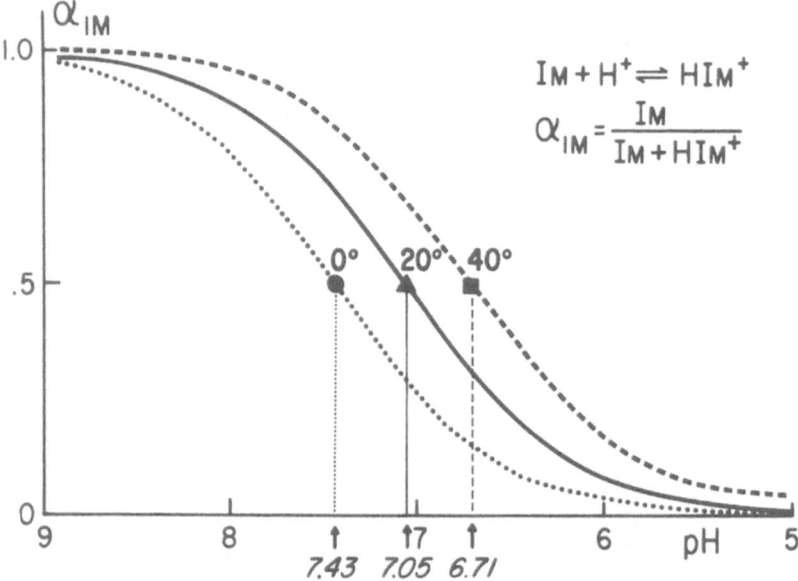

Fig. 5. Titration curve for peptide-linked histidyl imidazole groups showing marked temperature dependence of pK_{Im}. Protein histidine imidazole groups are considered to be characterized by a single pK_{Im} and a $\Delta H°$ of 7 kCal/mol for computation of α_{Im}. pK_{Im} values are indicated for 0°, 20° and 40°.

bicarbonate concentration with increasing P_{CO_2} arises from titration of protein histidine imidazole by carbonic acid, viz.,

$$H_2CO_3 + Im = HCO_3^- + HIm^+.$$

The titration curve for histidine imidazole is depicted in the upper panel. Three points along the CO_2 combining curve are indicated; lines connecting each point through the origin are pH isopleths. The pH isopleths have been visually connected to the corresponding point along the pH abscissa of the imidazole titration plot above. As CO_2 partial pressure increases and pH decreases, α_{Im} falls as more imidazole groups bind a proton and change their charge state from 0 to +1. Note that titration of protein by CO_2 can *only* occur with a change in α. When α is unchanged, on the other hand, bicarbonate is neither produced nor consumed.

Role of temperature in CO_2-protein interactions

If temperature is now permitted to change we observe the behavior depicted in Fig. 7. The CO_2 combining curve of normal whole blood, shown in the lower left panel, is very sensitive to temperature variation [5]. Note the points at which the combining curves for 0°, 20° and 40° are intersected when the P_{CO_2} is 7 torr; blood at zero degrees contains about three times as much CO_2 as it does at 40°. This large

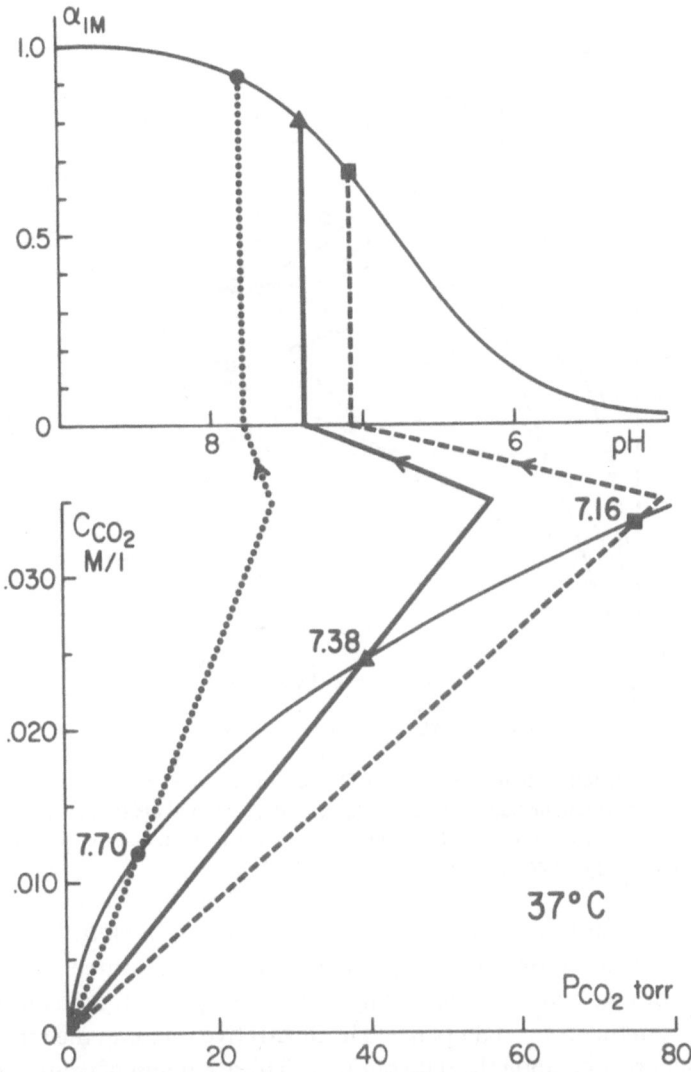

Fig. 6. Carbon dioxide combining curve of human whole blood (lower panel) and titration curve of protein histidine imidazole groups (upper panel). The diagonal straight lines in the lower graph are constant pH isopleths; these isopleths have been connected by straight line segments to the corresponding pH values on the abscissa of the titration curve.

difference is principally due to the increase in the histidine imidazole pK_{Im} signifying the binding of more protons at lower temperature, creating thereby more bicarbonate. If now we simulate change of temperature in vivo and compare blood changing temperature at constant CO_2 content (line at $C_{CO_2} = 24$ mM/1 in Fig. 7 lower left) we find that line intersects the CO_2 combining curves at successively lower CO_2 partial pressures as temperature falls. Isopleths of constant pH through the same intersection points are visually connected to the pH

22

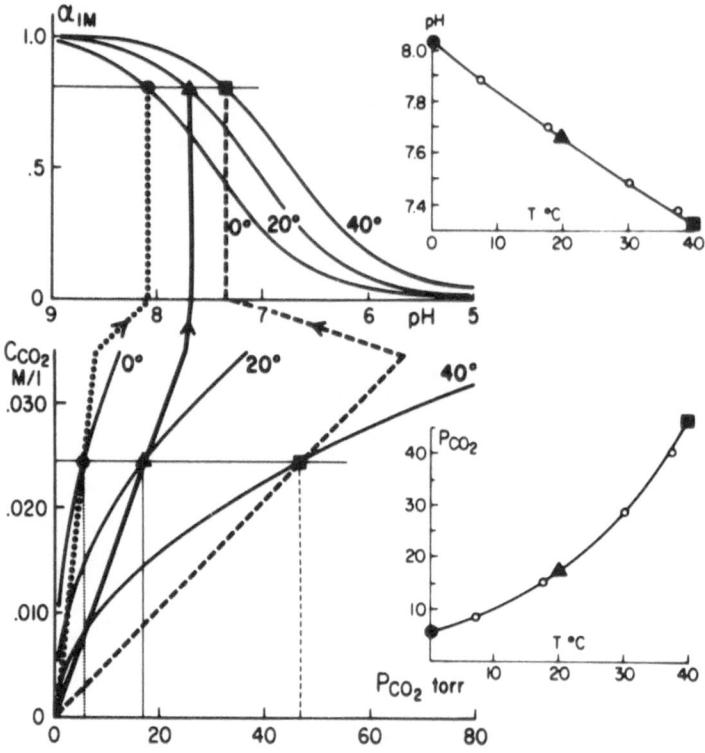

Fig. 7. The effect of temperature on (a) the CO_2 combining curves of blood (lower left), (b) the titration curves for protein histidine imidazole (upper left), (c) blood pH (upper right) and (d) blood CO_2 partial pressure (lower right). The effects of change in temperature at constant P_{CO_2} are diagrammed for α_{Im}, pH, and P_{CO_2}.

abscissa of the histidine imidazole titration plot in the upper left. These pH values at 0°, 20° and 40° are shown directly plotted against temperature in the panel in the upper right of Fig. 7; the corresponding CO_2 partial pressures are plotted against temperature in the lower right panel. The illustrative points at the three temperatures are superposed upon the data of Fig. 2. The argument of central importance in Fig. 7 is that α_{Im} (upper left panel) *does not change with temperature* under these conditions. Unlike the isothermal (37°) case presented in Fig. 6, when pH and P_{CO_2} change solely due to temperature variation of blood at constant gas content, no titration of the protein occurs, and alpha remains constant.

Importance of constant alpha to erythrocyte function

The utility to cell function of preserving alpha imidazole as temperature changes can be seen by observing red cell volume and ionic composition under these conditions. Erythrocytes by virtue of their large water and anion permeabilities are well known to change volume and ion composition when their intracellular hemoglobin is titrated either by varying CO_2 tension or by addition of fixed acid or base to plasma. Figure 8 illustrates the consequences of reducing carbon dioxide tension *at constant temperature,* thereby titrating intraerythrocyte protein. As plasma pH increases, both red cell volume and the ratio of chloride ion concentrations in red cell water to plasma water (r_{Cl}) diminish. Chloride is a convenient anion to measure because its Donnan concentration ratio is readily followed using [36]Cl; chloride is, however, equally useful as a marker for following the other two important permeable anions of this system, bicarbonate and hydroxyl ions. As plasma pH increases the concentration of permeable anions in cell water decreases because the net negative charge on hemoglobin increases. Intracellular protein's net negative charge is altered when histidyl imidazole

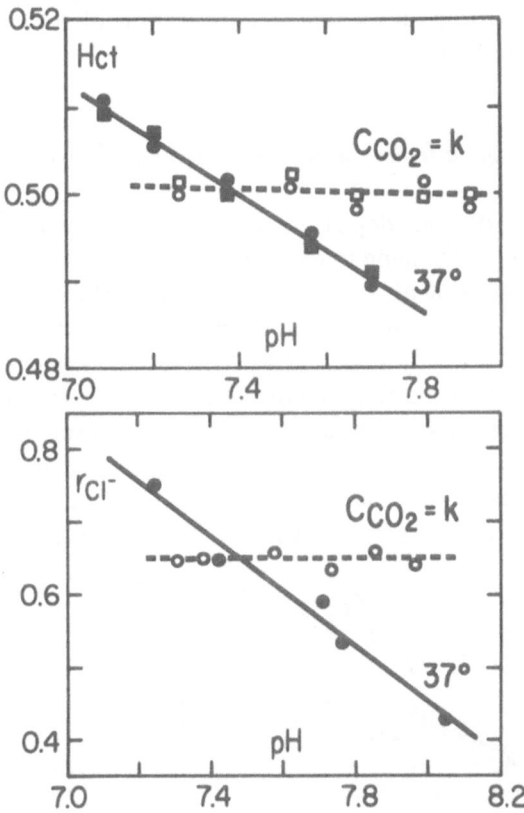

Fig. 8. The effect of changing pH on red cell volume measured as hematocrit ratio (above) and on the Donnan distribution of chloride ions (below). The ratio of chloride ion concentration (MEq/liter water) intracellularly to plasma chloride concentration is defined as the Donnan chloride ratio $[r_{Cl} = (Cl^-)_c/(Cl^-)_p]$. Plasma pH, plotted on the abscissa, was varied in two ways: At a constant temperature of 37° C, the partial pressure of CO_2 was varied (isothermal pH variation); in the second method, plasma pH of blood of constant gas content was altered only by changing temperature (constant P_{CO_2}).

groups lose their proton and positive unit charge, and thereby become uncharged. Alpha imidazole therefore increases. Decrease in the intracellular concentration of permeable anions means loss of osmotic equivalents; water thereby leaves the red cell resulting in a decrease in red cell volume.

Contrast the effect on these properties of changing plasma pH (and P_{CO_2}) by *altering only the temperature* at constant CO_2 content. Under these circumstances there is no change in red cell hemoglobin alpha imidazole, hence there is neither change in protein net charge, intraerythrocyte anion concentration, nor water content (see Fig. 8). By keeping a constant alpha imidazole as temperature changes, the red cell preserves its composition and volume independent of temperature. Thus in the body red cells rapidly change temperature in arteries and veins, but can do so under conditions that safeguard cell volume and ion distribution. Conservation of ion concentrations and cell volume whatever the operating temperature is an elegant demonstration of the practical utility of alphastat regulation in vivo.

Responses to a change in temperature at constant gas content: Summary

A symbol and arrow diagram depicting relationships between the physical chemical variables for blood changing temperature at constant gas content is shown in Fig. 9. Histidine-imidazole pK_{Im} changes inversely (dashed arrow) with temperature variation, the independent variable. Because blood and tissue are overwhelmingly protein buffer systems, the pH change is in the same direction (solid arrow) and magnitude as the pK_{Im} change. Since the difference ($pH - pK_{Im}$) stays constant in well buffered solutions like blood and cytoplasm, α_{Im} does not change. Z, the net charge on the protein, is invariant since the fraction of histidine-imidazole groups bearing a +1 charge ($1 - \alpha_{Im}$) is unchanged. The carbonic acid/bicarbonate equilibrium responds to the pH change with an altered CO_2 partial

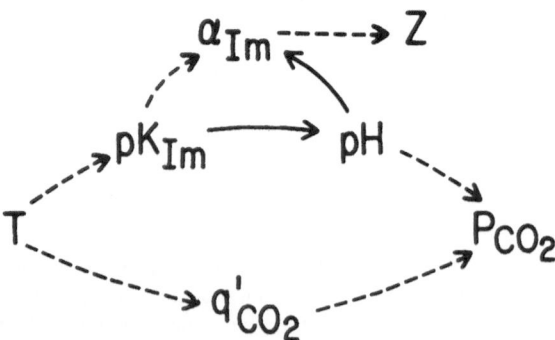

Fig. 9. Symbol and arrow diagram depicting relationship between acid-base parameters for blood changing temperature at constant gas content. Solid arrows denote a direct, dashed arrows an inverse, relationship between connected parameters.

pressure; pH and P_{CO_2} vary inversely. Note that temperature also has an inverse effect on CO_2 solubility (q'_{CO_2}); lowering temperature increases solubility. Quantitatively, however, this is a second order effect and can be ignored in qualitative discussion.

Let us now review the changes that occur in blood and tissue changing temperature at constant CO_2 content, like 37° blood leaving core to perfuse a cooled extremity. When temperature falls, pH increases and P_{CO_2} decreases significantly; normal acid-base status is not that of a pH-stat when temperature inhomogeneities exist in the system. The variable that remains constant is α_{Im}, and because of this invariance, the net charge on proteins is protected from change.

Inasmuch as there is no titration of protein even though pH and P_{CO_2} change significantly, CO_2 stores are neither increased nor decreased as blood or tissue temperature alters. The concentration of bicarbonate ion does not change. This stability obviates any need to load or unload CO_2 stores as temperature changes; if constant pH were required in changing temperature, CO_2 from metabolism would have to be loaded as temperature decreased. If CO_2 stores changed whenever a tissue changed temperature, a time lag would occur in establishing normal acid-base conditions arising from the need to wait for metabolism to provide the additional CO_2 or for perfusion to wash out the excess. By operating always at constant alpha, the transition from one regulated acid-base state to another on changing tissue temperature is instantly achieved. The conserved parameter that distinguishes temperature-invariant normal acid-base status is α_{Im}; this type of acid-base status regulation has been termed *alphastat* control [5, 6]. In the case of regional temperature variation alphastat control is a purely physical chemical property of the protein buffered aqueous solution; however whole body alphastat control requires full participation of all active physiological regulatory processes: ventilatory control of P_{CO_2}, renal control of plasma strong ion (buffer base) concentrations, and cell membrane strong ion pumps.

Lessons from animals of variable body temperature

For lower vertebrate classes that do not regulate body temperature directly as do homeothermic vertebrates, acid-base balance regulatory behavior is only recently well understood [5, 6, 7, 8]. Their acid-base regulation typifies alphastat control of open, metabolizing systems. In air-breathers among these groups, ventilatory control establishes precisely the required blood/tissue P_{CO_2} at each body temperature so that α_{Im} is maintained constant. Nonetheless, the carbon dioxide content of blood and tissues is unchanged; for an animal to change body temperature, no alteration in gas stores need occur to achieve a new regulated acid-base state. Thus air-breathers can change body temperature quickly and have large temperature gradients within the body and suffer neither transients nor hysteresis effects with respect to their acid-base state.

26

Water-breathers, on the other hand, so dedicate gill ventilation to oxygen extraction that they cannot afford to adjust carbon dioxide tension by changing of ventilation. Their mode of acid-base regulation is active transport of strong ions across gill epithelia. In order to maintain a constant alpha imidazole as their body temperature is lowered, they must take up strong base cations (buffer base) from their environment and load their carbon dioxide stores. On re-warming, these ion equivalents must be lost along with a portion of their carbon dioxide stores. This process involves many hours and is energetically costly. This approach to acid-base control is unavoidably associated with long transient imbalance states.

Figure 10 graphically summarizes the control of acid-base balance based on data from a large number of ectothermic vertebrates, both air- and water-breathers: fishes, amphibians and reptiles. In these classes $\alpha_{Im} = 0.8$ in whole blood independent of body temperature. This means that the actively regulated blood pH (to maintain $(pH - pK_{Im})$ constant) is different at each body temperature. In general these regulatory features may be viewed as mechanisms that permit a species to change body temperature without changing protein net charge state.

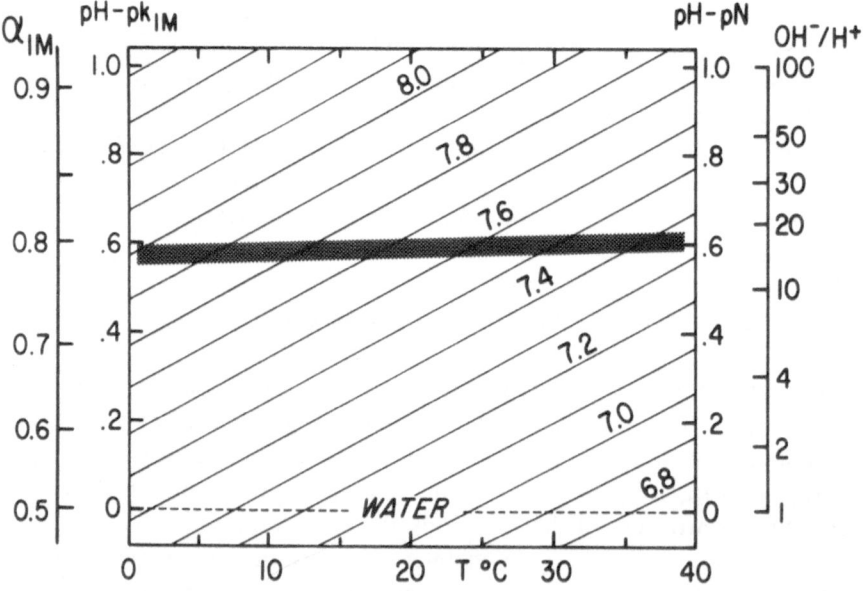

Fig. 10. Blood values for vertebrates including man as a function of temperature plotted on the left ordinate as the difference between blood pH and the pK of the histidyl imidazole group (or alpha imidazole) and on the right as the difference between blood pH and the pH of neutrality for water $(pH - pN)$ (or corresponding $(OH^-)/(H^+)$ ratio).

Alphastat control of ventilation

Air-breathing ectothermic vertebrates adjust their blood acid-base balance as body temperature changes by modifying ventilation rather than by renal adjustments in strong ions (buffer base). How is the correct ventilation achieved at each body temperature to establish the precise carbon dioxide partial pressure required to keep alpha imidazole constant? One mechanism by which this result can be attained assumes that the central chemoreceptors regulating ventilation and responsive to cerebrospinal fluid (CSF) pH are themselves histidyl imidazole groups. Brainstem chemoreceptor neurons are posited to have proton-sensitive proteins that progressively stimulate ventilation as alpha imidazole falls (protonation) below a certain set-point; these receptors silence respiratory efforts when deprotonation causes alpha to exceed the setpoint. Evidence in favor of this hypothesis derives from the effect on ventilation of ventricular perfusion with mock CSF solutions of varying pH. In a typical homeothermic mammal like the goat, relatively small increments in CSF hydrogen activity have a powerful stimulatory effect on ventilation [10]. Increments in hydrogen ion activity during CSF perfusion in an ectothermic vertebrate like a turtle shows an analogous effect, except that the ventilatory responce curve shifts when body temperature changes as shown in Fig. 11 [11]. If now the relative ventilation data for the goat at 37 degrees and for the turtle at two body temperatures are plotted against alpha imidazole (see Fig. 12), the data fall on a single curve [11]. This example indicates that by controlling alpha at a single histidyl imidazole site (the chemoreceptor neuron) carbon dioxide tension is established required to set alpha for all histidyl imidazole moieties wherever they occur in the proteins of the body. Note too, that when alphastat regulation is examined at one temperature only, as in man at 37° C, pH appears to be the regulated variable. Only when variable body temperature is employed is the regulation of imidazole protonation state apparent.

Relationships between alpha imidazole and relative alkalinity

Once earlier investigators had established that neither pH nor carbon dioxide tension is kept constant in closed or open systems as temperature varies the identity of the regulated parameter became the focus of analysis. Howell *et al.* [7] proposed that a property related to the dissociation of water, viz.

$$H_2O = H^+ + OH^-,$$

relative alkalinity, is conserved. Relative alkalinity refers to the ratio

$$(OH^-)/(H^+);$$

when $(OH^-) = -(H^+)$, neutrality obtains. Relative alkalinity can be related to the solution pH and to the negative logarithm of the dissociation constant of water (pKw) by

28

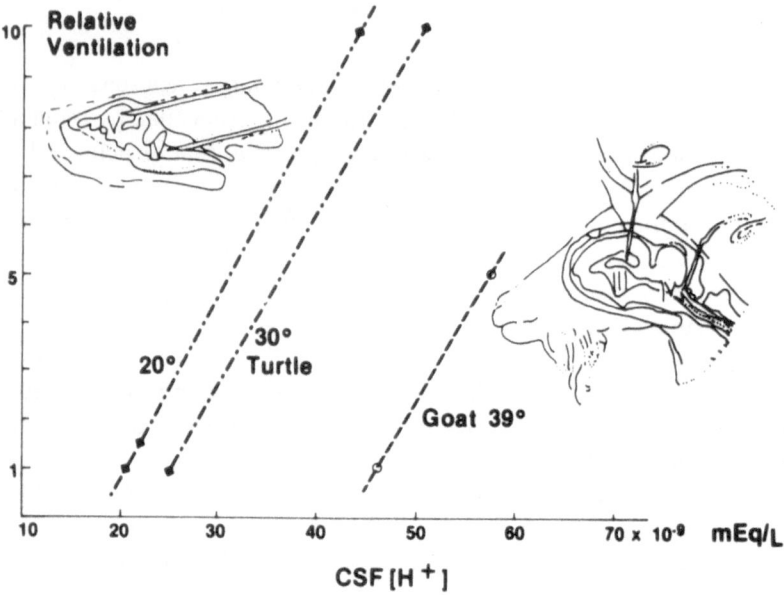

Fig. 11. Changes in relative ventilation plotted against CSF hydrogen ion concentratin during ventricular perfusion for the turtle *(Pseudemys)* at two different body temperatures and the goat at 39° C.

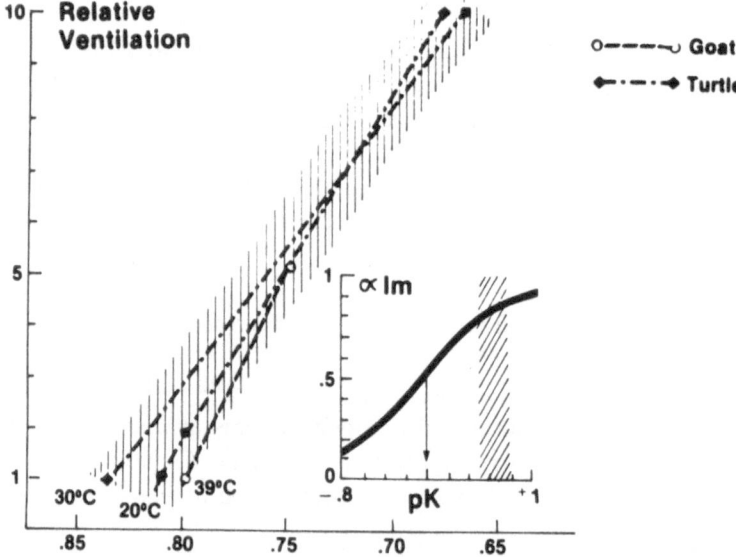

Fig. 12. Changes in relative ventilation during ventricular perfusion for turtles at two different body
temperatures, and goats at 39° C, plotted as a function of alpha imidazole. Hatched area indicates that
change in ventilation is a single-valued function of alpha imidazole despite temperature and species
differences. Insert: Alpha imidazole is plotted against the difference between the pH of mock CSF
perfusates minus the pK of histidyl imidazole (temperature corrected). Hatched area demonstrates
small changes in alpha required to cover full ventilatory range.

$$(OH^-)/(H^+) = 10^{(2pH - pKw)};$$

constant relative alkalinity requires that the exponent be unchanged as temperature varies, viz.,

$$2\ pH - pKw = k,$$

or, since 1/2 pKw is the pH of neutrality (pN), that

$$pH - 1/2pKw = pH - pN = k/2.$$

Thus constant relative alkalinity simply means that a constant ΔpH above neutrality is maintained (see Fig. 10).

Temperature significantly alters Kw and, therefore, the pH of neutrality. Since enthalpy of the dissociation of water is $14\ kcal\ mol^{-1}$ [9], the enthalpy for neutrality is half that, or $7\ kcal\ mol^{-1}$. This magnitude implies that constant relative alkalinity can only be achieved if pH changes with temperature at a rate of circa $-0.015\ \mu/^\circ C$.

Most physiological systems so far studied change pH on varying temperature at this rate, a rate equally consistent with description as constant relative alkalinity or constant alpha imidazole. Although these two ways of describing system behavior are frequently used interchangeably, one important difference between them deserves mention. When the appropriate acid-base equilibrium and conservation equations for well buffered protein systems are written, water's contribution to overall system acid-base behavior is seen to be several orders of magnitude too small to have a significant effect. With protein buffer values as high as encountered in blood and cytoplasm, the contribution of water's enthapy of dissociation to the behavior of the physical chemical acid-base temperature behavior is nil. For this reason use of alpha imidazole to relative alkalinity appears preferable in describing these systems. Moreover, although the effects of protonation of imidazole groups of protein histidyl residues on protein function are known for scores of detailed examples, a biochemical property specifically responsive to $(OH^-)/(H^+)$ has yet to be described.

Advantages of alphastat regulation of acid-base state

Inclusion of temperature in studies of acid-base regulation emphasizes the pervasive purpose of these processes, the preservation and optimization of the environment for protein function. Since histidine is the only titratable amino acid in proteins in the physiological pH range, and histidine-imidazolium groups can have a charge state of either 0 or +1, control of α_{Im} keeps protein net charge constant. Histidine charge state plays a central role as a determinant of protein tertiary and quaternary structure. Enzymological activity, cooperativity, and allosteric control are all dependent on conformation; hence, maintainance of a temperature-independent protein structure confers obbvious advantages both to the ectothermic vertebrate as well as to a mammal like man with a variety of tissue temperatures. Moreover, histidine is the most common amino acid found in the active site of enzymes where it functions as a base catalyst. Such function requires that the imidazole group be kept partially protonated, i.e. intracellular α_{Im} must be maintained somewhere about mid-range ($\alpha_{Im} = 0.5$) for optimal enzyme activity. At 37° C an alpha imidazole of 0.5 is found at a pH of 7.0–7.2, the range of values usually found in studies of intracellular pH. To facilitate preservation of the intracellular alpha, and to preserve a sink for diffusable weak acid metabolic end-products like lactic acid, it is necessary to maintain extracellular pH alkaline by about 0.2 units. Hence for alphastat control of the cytoplasmic space for protein function, an extracellular pH of 7.4 is required. Alphastat control of acid-base balance achieves this optimization not only at normal body temperature, but at any working tissue temperature.

Intracellular acid-base regulation

If acid-base regulation subserves the preservation of ionization state of protein histidyl imidazole groups, the ultimate focus of all acid-base regulation must be directed toward the intracellular compartment, the principal site of protein enzymatic activity. The linkage between intracellular and extracellular acid-base regulation is not as yet well understood as it must operate in vivo. Experimental studies have for analytial convenience tended to uncouple the two phases. Significant studies have addressed the participation of intracellular processes in defending against a generalized extracellular acidosis or alkalosis. However, the apposite situation physiologically is surely the role an extracellular regulated state plays in facilitating intracellular preservation of acid-base state during metabolic activity that provokes a severe intracellular acid-base perturbation.

Research of the past 15 years has demonstrated that intracellular acid-base regulation is a non-equilibrium steady-state dependent upon active acid extrusion mechanisms in the cell membrane [13]. These mechanisms are most frequently found to involve separate, or combined, cation or anion antiports: furosemide-sensitive proton for sodium ion exchange, and disulfonic acid stilbene derivative sensitive chloride for bicarbonate ion exchange. The range of regulated pH_i values reported in mammals at 37° C is 6.9–7.1, i.e. a pH_i range that fixes alpha imidazole at about 0.5, precisely the mid-titration range required for optimizing histidyl imidazole participation in catalyzed reactions. Alphastat control of the extracellular compartment may play an important role in stabilizing extracellular substrate concentrations for the acid extrusion transport protein (i.e. extracellular [HCO_3]), in setting tissue CO_2 partial pressure, as well as in adjusting the regulated pH_i set-point as temperature varies. Investigations to determine how the regulated set-point for pH_i varies as body temperature changes are only now in progress. Data from mammalian systems are as yet lacking; however, data from non-mammalian air- and water-breathing vertebrates showing that change in regulated pH$_i$ set-point follows an alphastat pattern have recently been reviewed [14].

Practical aspects of acid-base management in hypothermia

Acid-base management of a patient experiencing general body hypothermia is greatly facilitated by the alphastat concept of acid-base regulation. Because of the underlying physical-chemical properties that result in blood pH and carbon dioxide pressure changes as temperature is varied at constant gas content, it is possible to learn all that one needs to know by examining the acid-base status of a blood sample at one temperature. If blood in a blood-gas apparatus measured at 37° C has normal acid-base characteristics, whatever the body temperature of the patient from whom the sample is taken, that blood will have a constant normal value for alpha imidazole at all temperatures. If however the sample reflects an altered CO_2 partial pressure, indicative of the loading or unloading CO_2 stores, ventilation can be changed to correct the imbalance. In practice continued use of the initial pre-cooling tidal volume and frequency will insure the required relative overventilation as body temperature falls and need only minimal further adjustment. Similarly, if the blood sample when measured at 37° C at a P_{CO_2} of 40 torr is seen to have a metabolic acidosis, that acidosis can be compensated for by the addition of isotonic sodium bicarbonate in the usual way. By managing the patient from an acid-base point of view as though he were at normal body temperature, an acid-base state of constant alpha imidazole can be achieved whatever the extent and duration of hypothermic excursion.

If on the other hand, the alternative is considered, i.e. correcting measured blood pH and P_{CO_2} values to body temperature in each instance, managemant becomes most complicated. First, simple 'Rosenthal blood temperature correction factors' [12] are not truly constant [2]; some means of determining the correct factor or application of a complex algorithm would be needed. This criticism also applies to the temperature correction for carbon dioxide tension.Secondly, a set of normal pH and P_{CO_2} values for each temperatue will be needed. Additionally, core temperature is frequently changing rapidly and tissue temperatures are not uniform when cooling or re-warming is in progress. Which temperature is used and how representative it is becomes important. Finally bicarbonate correction for fixed acid loads under a temperature-correction scheme of management is seriously hampered by lack of appropriate nomograms for temperatures other than 37° C.

Conclusion

Is alphastat regulation of acid-base balance appropriate for acutely hypothermic human patients? Our answer is affirmative for four reasons: (1) Alphastat regulation of acid-base balance is a common homeostatic pattern seen throughout vertebrate evolution; (2) The fundamental elements of this regulation are still apparent in normal man when tissues temperatures depart from core temperature; (3) The significance to tissue and cell function of alphastat control is evident; and (4) Alphastat principles facilitate ready analysis and correction of acid-base disturbances at all temperatures.

References

1. Bazett HC,Love L, Newton M, Eisenberg L, Day R, Forster R: Temperature changes in blood flowing in arteries and veins in man. J Appl Physiol 1: 3–19, 1948.
2. Reeves RB: Temperature-induced changes in blood acid-base status: pH and P_{CO_2} in a binary buffer. J Appl Physiol 40: 752–761, 1976.
3. Reeves RB: Temperature-induced changes in blood acid-base status: Donnan r_{Cl} and red cell volume. J Appl Physiol 40: 762–767, 1976.
4. Matthew JB, Hanania G, Gurd FRN: Electrostatic effects in hemoglobin: hydrogen ion equilibria in human deoxy- and oxyhemoglobin A. Biochemistry 18: 1919–1927, 1979.
5. Reeves RB, Rahn H: Patterns in vertebrate acid-base regulation. In: Evolution of Respiratory Processes: A Comparative Approach, Wood S and Lenfant C (eds). Dekker, N.Y.: 225–252.
6. Reeves RB: An imidazole alphastat hypothesis for vertebrate acid-base regulation: tissue carbon dioxide content and body temperature in bullfrogs. Respir. Physiol. 14: 219–236, 1972.
7. Howell BJ, Baumgardner F, Bondi K, Rahn H: Acid-base balance in cold-blooded vertebrates as a function of body temperature. Am. J. Physiol. 218: 600–606, 1970.
8. Reeves RB: The interaction of body temperature and acid-base balance in ectothermic vertebrates. Ann. Rev. Physiol. 39: 559–586, 1977.
9. Robinson RA, Stokes RH: Electrolyte Solutions. London, Butterworths, Appendix 12.2, p. 544.
10. Pappenheimer JR, Fencl V, Heisey S, Held D: Role of cerebral fluids in control of respiration as studied in unanesthetized goats. Am. J. Physiol. 208: 436–450, 1965.
11. Hitzig BM: Temperature-induced changes in turtle CSF pH and central control of ventilation. Respir. Physiol. 49: 205–222, 1982.
12. Rosenthal TB: The effect of temperature on the pH of blood and plasma in vitro J. Biol. Chem. 173: 25–30, 1948.
13. Roos A, Boron WF: Intracellular pH. Physiol. Rev. 61: 296–434, 1981.
14. Reeves RB: Alphastat regulation of intracellular acid–base state? Proc. 1st. Int. Congr. Comp. Physiol. Biochem. (in press).

3. Acid-base regulation during hibernation

A. MALAN

Abstract

The 'constant pH' strategy of hibernators involves loading considerable amounts of CO_2 during the entrance into hibernation, and hyperventilating to eliminate this CO_2 during the arousal. Together with the decrease of blood alpha imidazole, this indicates that the blood pH and P_{CO_2} observed in hibernation result from the combined effects of a respiratory acidosis and a change in temperature. The respiratory acidosis also affects most intracellular compartments of the body, except for the heart and liver, in which a metabolic compensation takes place, resulting in a nearly constant alpha imidazole. Respiratory acidosis exerts inhibitory influences on various nervous and metabolic processes, and probably contributes to the great amplitude of regulation of metabolic rate characteristic of hibernation. The inhibition would be at least partly removed early in the arousal by hyperventilation, while during deep hibernation heart and liver would be protected by the alphastat control of intracellular pH. Our ignorance of the mechanisms ensuring the selective inhibition or facilitation of pHi regulation according to tissues precludes the clinical application of the hibernation model.

Introduction

Hibernating mammals spontaneously undergo deep hypothermia (body temperature lower than 10° C) with a nearly 100% rate of recovery. This is quite exceptional in warm-blooded animals, and it is therefore tempting to try to imitate the hibernator when hypothermia is to be artificially induced in man for surgical purposes. In particular, when body temperature is lowered, the hibernator does not increase blood pH according to the imidazole alphastat rule, but rather tends to keep a constant pH. Should the same be done in hypothermia in human patients? To answer this question, one needs to know whether the pH–temperature relationship of hibernators is directly dictated by hypothermia, or if this acidotic deviation from the general alphastat rule plays any definite role in the physiology of hibernation. Before analyzing hibernation acid-base phenomena, let us recall some important characteristics of hibernation, to which they may be related.

General features of natural hibernation

Surviving a cold winter

Hibernation is found in many orders of mammals, from the most primitive such as the echidna to small primates such as the lemur. Its most typical representatives are rodents (e.g. marmots, ground squirrels, hamsters) and bats living in the temperate and subarctic zones of the Northern Hemisphere [1]. Hibernation has most probably evolved as an adaptation to the scarcity of food in winter. Reducing body temperature by 10° C reduces the resting energy requirements by a factor of about 2.2. By lowering its body temperature from 37° C to 7° C, for example, a hibernator will thus reduce its nutritional needs by a factor of 2.2^3 or 10.7. The actual reduction factor is still higher, about 30 [2], which has led to the supposition that other inhibitory factors intervene in addition to temperature ([3] see below). Since the need for cold thermogenesis has also disappeared, the energy saving to be expected approximates 97% of normothermic resting metabolic rate. The actual economy is only about 88–90%, due to the cost of the periodic arousals [4, 5], but this is still enough to allow the animal to survive the whole winter on the food gathered during the preceding summer. In most species, this is stored as body fat, making up to 50% of body mass by the end of the summer [4]; only a few species such as the hamsters store food as such. A typical hibernator, the Richardson's ground squirrel, Citellus richardsonii, settles in a burrow in the fall after a suitable endocrine and fattening preparation, and then starts a cycling pattern of body temperature, Tb, in which bouts of deep hibernation with Tb less than 3° C above ambient temperature, lasting 3 to 19 days, alternate with short arousals (Fig. 1). During an arousal, the animal spontaneously rewarms back to a Tb of 37° C within 2 to 6 hours, and stays normothermic for 5 to 24 hours before returning to hibernation [5]. Similar patterns are found in the other species. Periodic arousals represent 83% of the total energy budget of the hibernation season in the Richardson's ground squirrel [5]. The reason why they are important enough to justify that expenditure is still unknown.

A controlled lowering of body temperature

By contrast with ectothermic (cold-blooded) animals in which changes of Tb are directly imposed by the variations of ambient temperature, the reduction of Tb in hibernation is a controlled and reversible phenomenon. In small mammals, thermal responses are largely controlled by the temperature of the preoptic area

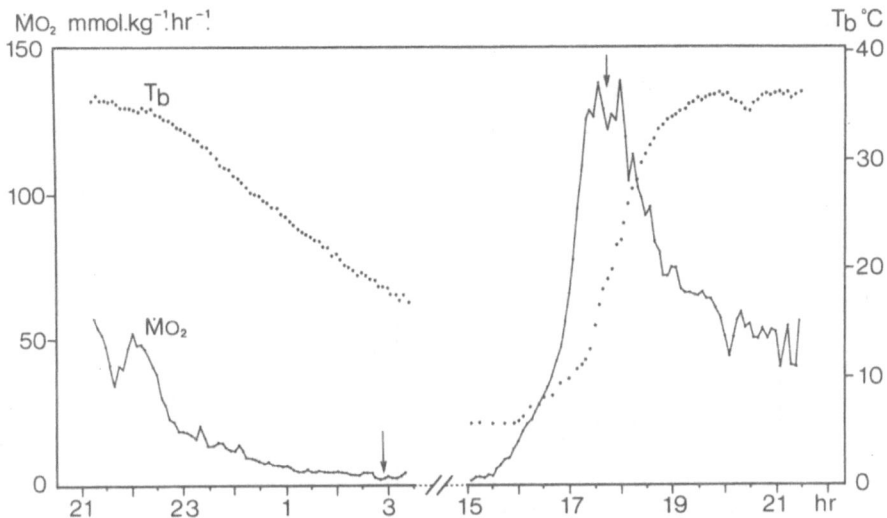

Fig. 1. Oxygen consumption, M_{O_2}, and brain temperature, Tb, of a Richardson's ground squirrel during entrance into hibernation (left) and arousal (right). Notice the 40:1 scope of metabolic rate for the same Tb of 18° C (arrows). Adapted from Wang [5].

of the anterior hypothalamus (POAH). This temperature can be manipulated, in normothermy or in hibernation, by means of chronically implanted water-perfused thermodes (Fig. 2) [6, 7, 8, 9]. During deep hibernation, a low preoptic area of the hypothalamus (POAH) temperature is maintained in the face of ambient changes by appropriate thermogenic or thermolytic mechanisms; compared to normothermy, the set temperature and the gain of the regulation are much reduced, but the pattern is very similar. From the point of view of temperature regulation, hibernation thus resembles a negative fever, both hibernation and fever corresponding to a resetting of the hypothalamic thermostat. As we will see below, the same kind of resetting probably occurs for acid-base regulation.

Functioning over a wide range of body temperature

Even though metabolic activity is reduced in deep hibernation, it is not completely suppressed, and at least a certain number of metabolic pathways and of physiological functions (circulation, ventilation, etc.) have to be kept in operation at a low Tb. Higher cortical activity is generally inhibited, only evoked potentials being visible on an otherwise flat EEG [10, 11]. But brainstem and limbic activity are maintained, and the animal will respond to tactile or auditory stimuli by initiating an arousal [12, 13]. Correspondingly, the seasonal preparation for hibernation involves biochemical changes typically found in ectothermic species which remain active over wide fluctuations of ambient temperature (eurythermal species). In particular, summer enzymes tailored for homeothermal

36

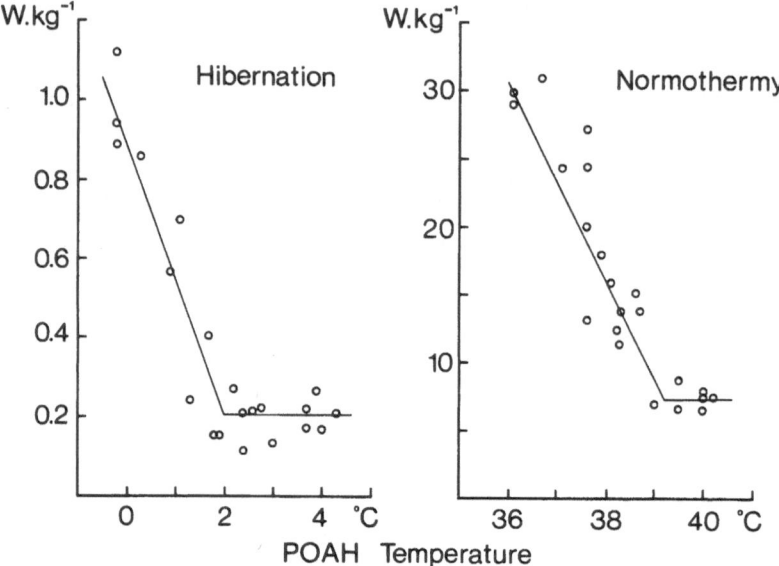

Fig. 2. Characteristics of hypothalamic temperature regulation for a golden-mantled ground squirrel during hibernation (left) and normothermy (right): metabolic rate (W.kg⁻¹) versus the temperature (°C) of the preoptic area of the hypothalamus (POAH). Regulation is conserved in hibernation, but the threshold for regulatory thermogenesis and the slope are reduced. Redrawn from Heller *et al.* [9].

operation are replaced by isozymes characterized by a nearly constant affinity for their substrates or modulators, and by a monotonic dependency of maximal reaction velocity on temperature, over the full 35–5°C temperature range [14, 15, 16, 17, 18, 19]. These features are adaptive for the conservation of metabolic regulation in the face of wide changes of Tb [18]. When the enzymes are pH-sensitive, this conservation requires an alphastat regulation of pH. This has been demonstrated for two important mammalian enzymes, the eurythermal isozyme of lactate dehydrogenase and the phosphofructokinase [20, 21].

Achieving a high flexibility of metabolic control

The hibernator differs from an ectothermic vertebrate in a very important respect, however. While most reptiles cannot increase their metabolic rate more than about six times the basal level at a given Tb [22], a mammalian hibernator can vary its oxygen consumption by a factor of at least 40:1 at the same body temperature (18°C), depending on whether this Tb is reached while arousing from, or entering into hibernation (Fig. 1) [3, 5]. This is twice as much as in best human athletic performances. Most probably, the hibernator does not achieve this high metabolic scope by increasing the energy output beyond the 'Olympic' level during the peak effort of arousal, but rather by reducing its metabolic rate below the so-called 'basal' metabolic rate when entering into, or staying in deep hibernation [3, 23]. Such a reduction is a characteristic of prolonged starvation in mammals and birds [24, 25]. Like a starving animal, the hibernating mammal has to supply most of its energy requirements from fat reserves, and to reduce to a minimum the utilization of glucose and proteins. But hibernation differs from starvation in that the transition times, from normal to depressed metabolism and back, are much shorter, especially during emergency arousal. Any inhibitory factor involved in metabolic depression has therefore to be quickly built up or eliminated.

Acid-base characteristics of hibernating mammals

The 'constant pH' of hibernators

When the arterial pH and P_{CO_2} of a hibernating mammal are measured with electrodes calibrated at the animal's body temperature, one most often gets results such as in Fig. 3: compared to the normothermic state, pH is constant or slightly increased, while P_{CO_2} is decreased. In some species, pH is increased in hibernation, but by far not to the extent observed in ectotherms for the same temperature decrease (Table 1).

By the same reasoning as for ectotherms (Chapter 2), these open system values of pH and P_{CO_2} result at each Tb from the steady state balance between the production and elimination of CO_2, metabolic acids, etc., and not from a passive

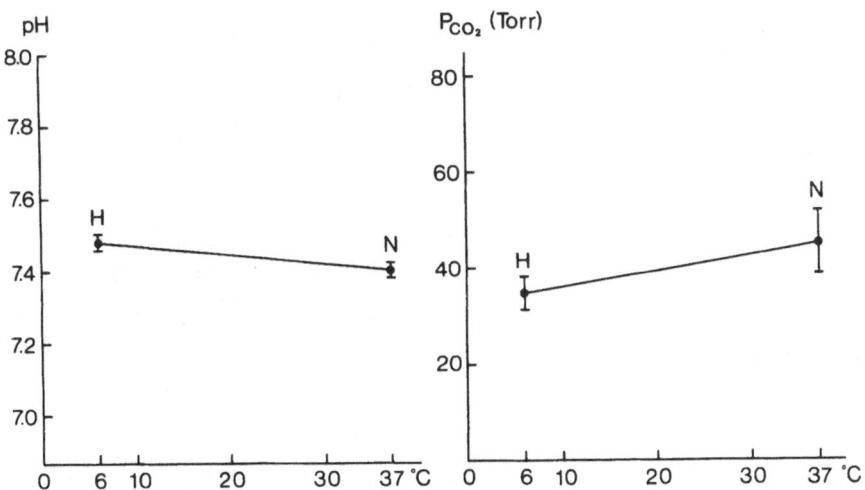

Fig. 3. Arterial pH and P_{CO_2} measured at body temperature in European hamsters, hibernating (H) or normothermic (N). Mean ± S.D. Compared to normothermy, pH is slightly increased in hibernation while P_{CO_2} is decreased. As a first approximation, both can be considered fairly constant.

effect of temperature. Increases of respiratory rate in response to breathing hypercapnic or hypoxic gas mixtures have been observed in hibernators [26, 27]. The range of spontaneous variability of blood pH and P_{CO_2} is within the same range in deep hibernation as in normothermy (Fig. 3, Table 1), indicating that at least the ventilatory homeostasis of these quantities is conserved.

Is this a homeostasis of pH?

As we have already seen, hibernation has evolved separately in various orders of

Table 1. Arterial pH and P_{CO_2} of hibernating or normothermic hibernators, measured at body temperature. Mean and S.D., or range.

	Body temperature (* = assumed) (°C)	pH	P_{CO_2} (Torr)	Ref.
A. HIBERNATING				
Hedgehog	5	7.45	30.1	68
	6*	7.46 (0.04)	26.5 (4.4)	69
Ground squirrel	5	7.39 (0.03)	35	70
	6	7.44 (0.03)	32.9 (2.3)	71
Alpine marmot	8	7.57 (0.03)	33.3 (3.4)	28
European hamster	9	7.57 (0.02)	36.1 (9.0)	28
	6	7.48 (0.02)	34.3 (2.5)	(†)
Golden hamster	6	7.46 (0.02)	40.5 (4.6)	73
Common dormouse	6	7.44 (0.03)	27.4 (2.6)	73
B. NORMOTHERMIC				
Hedgehog	32	7.38 (7.29–7.51)	43.6 (31.9–55.0)	68
	36*	7.33 (0.03)	53.5 (3.3)	69
Ground squirrel	37	7.39 (0.06)	42	70
	37	7.40 (0.03)	47.7 (5.0)	71
Marmot (2 species)	35.8	7.49 (0.02)	30	72
European hamster	37	7.40 (0.02)	45.3 (6.6)	28
Golden hamster	37*	7.30 (0.02)	59.7 (1.7)	73

* Malan, unpublished

mammals. It is therefore quite recent in terms of biochemical evolution, so that only slight changes may have occurred at the molecular level. There should be no fundamental difference in the general biochemical organization of hibernators compared to other mammals and to reptiles. This applies to the buffers and to the acid-base regulating systems in general. Thus the pH and P_{CO_2} vs. temperature relationships of blood in vitro are the same as those described by Reeves (Chapter 2) in ectothermic, nonhibernating mammals [28]. More striking, when the diurnal ground squirrel of the deserts of California, Spermophilus tereticaudus, reverts to heat storage behavior like a camel and lets its body temperature fluctuate between 30 and 42° C to reduce evaporative water loss, blood pH and P_{CO_2} are regulated according to the constant alpha strategy as observed in amphibians and reptiles. However, in the same animal, when the Tb fluctuations are associated with torpor, a constant pH is found, as is typical in the mammalian hibernator [29]. The constant pH strategy is, therefore, not imposed by biochemical peculiarities of mammals.

The biochemical similarity between the animals which adopt the constant pH tactics and those which favor the constant alpha can be extended to the pH metering systems of the organism. The mechanisms which regulate intracellular pH in nerve and muscle cells of crayfish (Fig 4) [30] and in hepatocytes of eels [31]

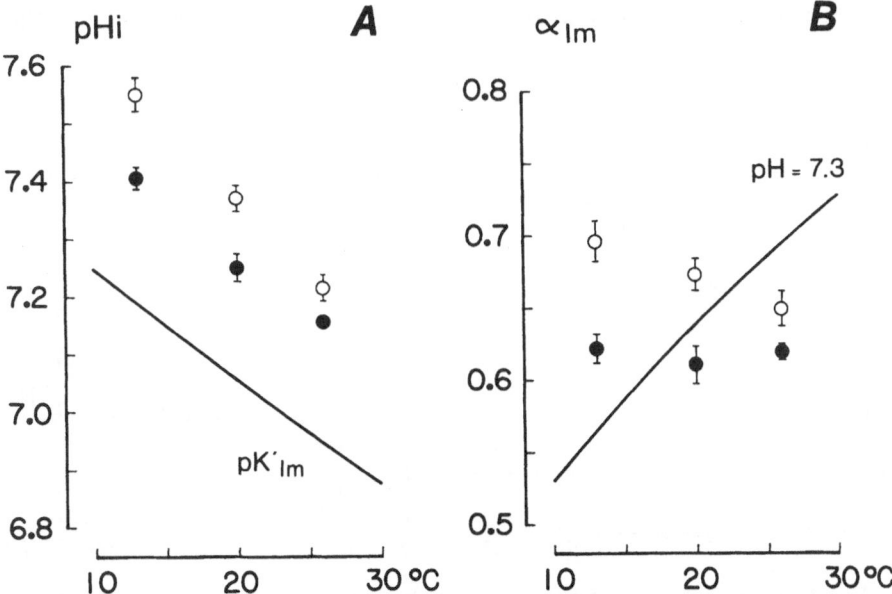

Fig. 4. Left panel: Intracellular (cytosolic) pH measured with microelectrodes in crayfish neurones (open symbols) and skeletal muscles (closed symbols). Solid line: protein imidazole pK'. Right panel: Same data expressed as the dissociation ratio of imidazole groups, alpha. Solid line: the variation of alpha with temperature if a constant pH of 7.3 is maintained. The membrane ionic exchange mechanisms which regulate intracellular pH at a given temperature keep a fairly stable alpha imidazole when temperature is varied. (Reproduced from Rodeau [30]).

40

as well as the medullary receptor involved in CSF pH regulation of turtles [32], all rely on the titration of protein imidazole (or imidazole-like) groups. Strictly speaking, they can be described as pH detectors only at a constant temperature, and should rather be termed alpha imidazole detectors. A mammal must be equally devoid of true pH detectors. Its carotid body and medullary receptors probably sense and regulate an alpha imidazole and not a pH, and this regulated alpha is shifted to the acid side in hibernation. In the same way as hibernation temperature regulation corresponds to the maintenance of a lower POAH temperature (see Fig. 2), hibernation acid-base regulation can be described as the maintenance of alpha at a reduced level.

The 'constant pH' requires loading CO_2

Is a hibernator's blood acidic only because the acidity sensor sees it that way, or because some acid has been added to the blood? A first answer is the following: since all the acid-base properties of mammalian blood in vitro [33, 34] apply to a hibernator's blood also, we can calculate [35, 33, 36] or experimentally determine what becomes of pH and P_{CO_2} as temperature is changed from 37 to 6° C or from 6 to 37° C, when no chemical substance (CO_2, acids, etc.) is added to or substracted from the blood, i.e. in closed system or 'anaerobic' conditions (Fig. 5). When

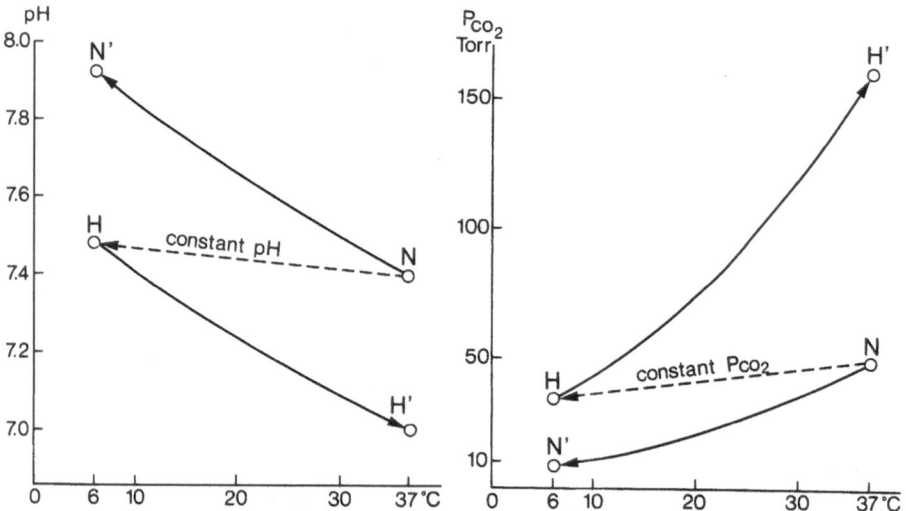

Fig. 5. Arterial pH and P_{CO_2} versus temperature relationships in the blood of a hibernator, the European hamster. H and N: in vivo data recorded on the same animal, as he went from hibernation (H) to normothermy (N) (same data as Fig. 8). Solid lines represent the evolution of pH or P_{CO_2} in closed-system (anaerobic) conditions in vitro, when temperature is either decreased from 37 to 6° C (N–N') starting from the normothermic condition, or increased from 6 to 37° C (H–H') starting from hibernation. The 'constant pH' and 'constant P_{CO_2}' in vivo transition cannot be achieved without chemical exchanges with the environment.

temperature decreases, blood pH increases mostly because protein imidazole is by far the predominant non-bicarbonate buffer, and because imidazole pK' increases as temperature is lowered [33, 34]. The decrease of P_{CO_2} when temperature decreases essentially results from a change in pK and an increase of CO_2 solubility. In these closed-system conditions, when the blood of a normothermic hamster (N, Fig. 5; data from the arousal of Fig. 8) with a pH of 7.40 and a P_{CO_2} of 49 Torr at 37° C is cooled to 6° C, it reaches a pH of 7.92 and a P_{CO_2} of 8.6 Torr (N'). Conversely, the blood from the same animal in hibernation (H) with a pH of 7.48 and a P_{CO_2} of 34 Torr at 6° C, reaches a pH of 7.01 and a P_{CO_2} of 160 Torr when warmed to 37° C (H'). The hibernator's pH and P_{CO_2} cannot be reached from the normothermic state by the sole effect of temperature.

The same models (here a more detailed one [37]), can be used to calculate what has to be done to maintain a constant pH of 7.40 (and a constant P_{CO_2} of 40 Torr) – and thus to offset the increase of CO_2 solubility and imidazole pK' – when lowering the temperature from 37 to 6° C (Fig. 6). To achieve this, total blood C_{CO_2} has to be increased 78%, from 21.8 to 38.8 mmol/l. Correspondingly, the Donnan ratio for chloride r_{Cl} increases from 0.650 to 0.818, while the hematocrit goes from 0.450 to 0.475, similar to a CO_2 titration at 37° C [34, 37, 38]. By all

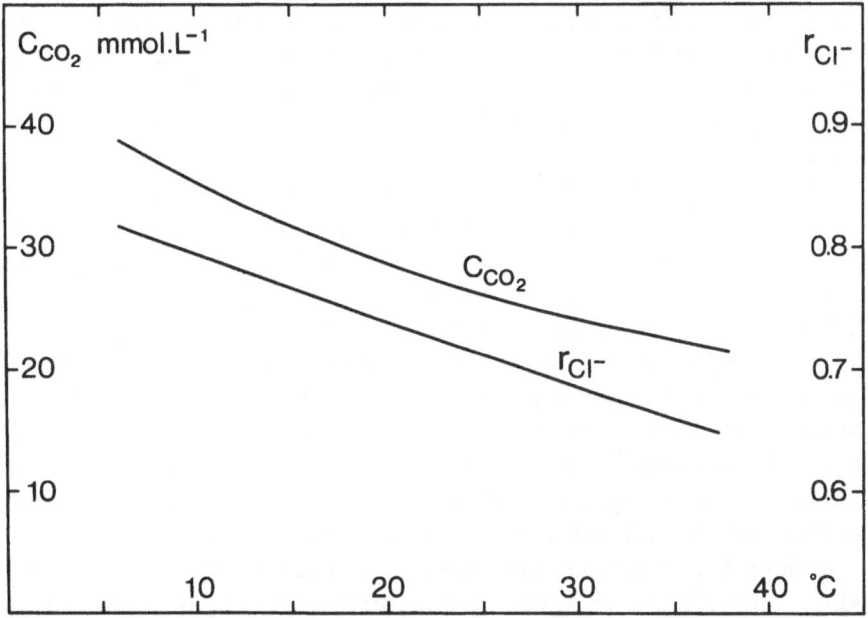

Fig. 6. *Upper curve:* Evolution of total blood CO_2 concentration required to keep a constant plasma pH of 7.40 and a P_{CO_2} of 40 Torr in mammalian blood when temperature is lowered from 37 to 6° C. *Lower curve:* The resulting evolution of the Donnan ratio for chloride distribution between plasma and red cells. In spite of the constancy of nominal values of plasma pH and P_{CO_2}, the Donnan ratio increases as temperature is lowered (and as C_{CO_2} is increased) like in a respiratory acidosis at 37° C.

these criteria, in order to keep a constant plasma pH when temperature is lowered a respiratory acidosis must be induced.

A representation of acid-base data at a variable temperature

Using such complex computer models is rather cumbersome and one needs a simpler, if more approximate way to estimate the amounts of CO_2, strong acids, etc. which have to be added to, or substracted from the blood in combination with the change in temperature to achieve a given acid-base change at a variable temperature. Since no chemical substance is exchanged with the environment when blood temperature is varied in closed (anerobic) conditions (Fig. 5), all the corresponding points along a pair of pH-temperature and P_{CO_2}-temperature curves correspond to chemically equivalent acid-base states, differing only by temperature. Let us then choose a standard temperature, say 37°C, at which all acid-base quantities will be expressed. By bringing a blood sample to 37°C in a closed syringe before reading pH and P_{CO_2}, one eliminates the effect of temperature and gets temperature-corrected values directly. The *corrected* pH, P_{CO_2}, and bicarbonate concentration, respectively pH*, $P^*_{CO_2}$ and $[HCO_3^-]^*$, can be plotted on a bicarbonate-pH diagram and analyzed in the classical way in terms of respiratory or metabolic disturbances, as if at a constant temperature of 37°C [36]. Instead of being directly measured, pH* and $P^*_{CO_2}$ can also be calculated using nomograms or computer models of acid-base versus temperature relationships [36, 37].

An important feature of this temperature correction procedure is that a constant pH* is nearly equivalent to a constant alpha imidazole. This results from blood buffer characteristics: as shown by Reeves [33, 34], plasma alpha imidazole remains nearly constant when blood temperature is varied in a closed system.

When compared with the normothermic data on a temperature-corrected bicarbonate-pH diagram (Fig. 7), the data from hibernating animals all show a large increase in $P^*_{CO_2}$, corresponding to the addition of CO_2 to the blood. The transition most often takes place along the in vivo titration curve of extracellular water, with a slope of 11.4 mEq.l^{-1}.pH unit^{-1} corresponding to blood equilibrated with interstitial fluid [39]. In a few instances, the data points lie above this buffer line, indicating the occurrence of a partial metabolic compensation of the respiratory acidosis. In all cases, hibernation is characterized by a very severe respiratory acidosis, with a decrease in pH* ranging from 0.24 to 0.48, whereas $P^*_{CO_2}$ is increased by a factor of 2.5 to 4.1.

The transition periods: entrance and arousal

Building up a respiratory acidosis during the entrance into hibernation requires a

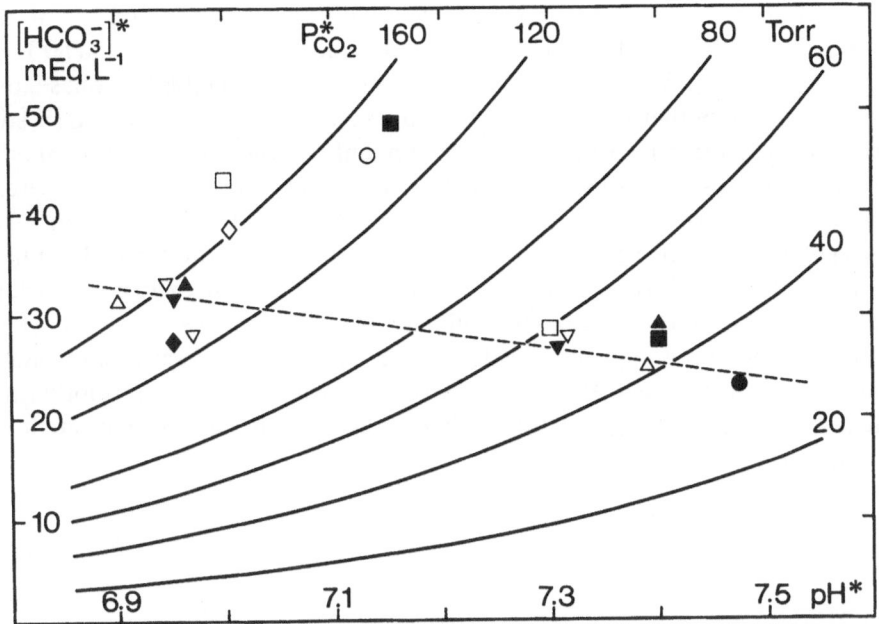

Fig. 7. Acid-base data of arterial blood of hibernators on a temperature-corrected bicarbonate-pH diagram. Standard temperature is 37°C. Broken line, buffer line of extracellular fluids, 11.4 mEq.l^{-1}.pH unit^{-1} [39]. Symbols: ▼, hedgehog [68]; ▽, id. [69]; △, ground squirrel [70]; ▲, id. [71]; ●, marmot [72]; ○, id. [28]; ◆, common dormouse [73]; ■, golden hamster [73]; □, European hamster [28]; ◇, id. (Malan, unpubl.). Compared with normothermy (right; P*$_{CO_2}$ 30–60 Torr), hibernation is characterized by a pronounced respiratory acidosis (left; P*$_{CO_2}$ 120–180 Torr), with some metabolic compensation in some species.

relative hypoventilation: as Tb goes down and as the animal progressively reduces its metabolic production of CO_2, the ventilatory flow rate has to be reduced still further. The opposite is true for the arousal.

Data are still nearly completely lacking for the entrance period. Snapp and Heller [40] have observed a temporary drop of the ventilatory gas exchange ratio ('respiratory quotient') at the beginning of the entrance phase in a ground squirrel, in agreement with the above predictions (cf also [74]).

The arousal phase is much better known. High gas exchange ratios (0.90 to 1.10) have long been observed during the initial phase of arousal [40, 41, 42]. This is unlikely to be due to switching from lipid to carbohydrate utilization, since during this early phase thermogenesis is of nonshivering origin and results mainly from lipid oxidation. More recently, ventilation could be measured together with oxygen consumption in hibernation and early arousal in marmots by whole body plethysmography [28]. The first overt physiological process in the arousal is a considerable hyperventilation. Without any change in breathing frequency at first, tidal volume increases by a factor of at least 2.5. This takes place before any rise in metabolic rate and tends therefore to deplete the accumulated CO_2 stores.

In the European hamster (Cricetus cricetus), over the first 45 to 60 min of the arousal, $P^*_{CO_2}$ falls from 162 ± 13 Torr to a value ranging between 60 and 80 Torr (Fig. 8; Malan, unpubl.), at least a twofold reduction. During this first phase, the rates of increase of thermogenesis and of Tb remain low (Fig. 1). Shivering is still absent, nonshivering heat being generated mainly by the abundant brown adipose tissue [43, 44]. Then a sharp increase in heat production takes place. Muscle shivering soon starts and heat production will peak while Tb is still less than 30° C (Fig.1) [4, 45, 44]. The accompanying lactate production accounts for about half the metabolic acidosis (Fig. 8). (The remaining could be due to extrusion of acidic equivalents from the cells for intracellular pH regulation – see below). Heat production then progressively subsides and the metabolic acidosis rapidly disappears. Later on, pH* and $P^*_{CO_2}$ progressively return toward the normothermic values (N; Fig. 8). A $P^*_{CO_2}$ less than 80 Torr thus seems to be a prerequisite for a powerful heat generation.

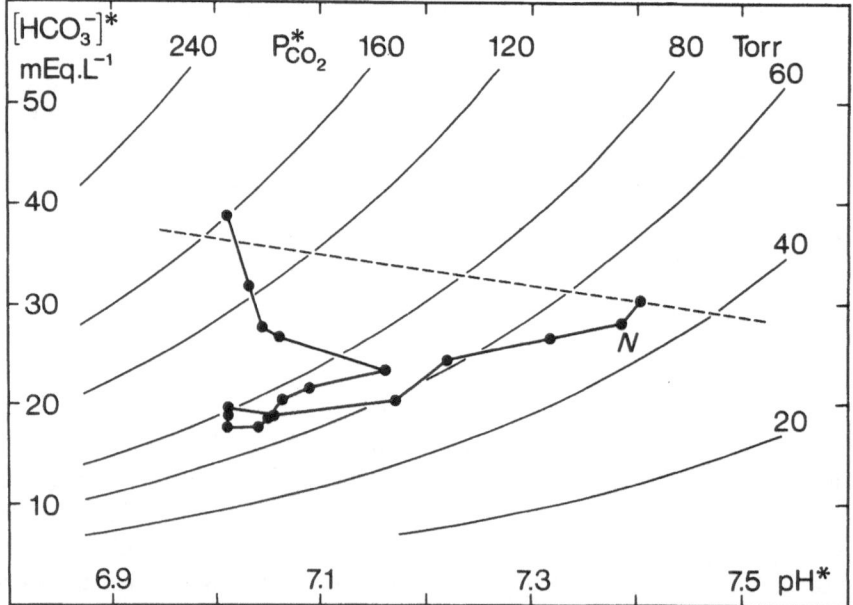

Fig. 8. Time-course of arterial acid-base variables in a European hamster arousing from hibernation. Temperature-corrected bicarbonate-pH diagram (standard temperature 37° C). Broken line, buffer line of extracellular fluids, 11.4 mEq.l^{-1}.pH unit^{-1} [39]. Sampling every 15 min. N: average of normothermic hamsters in winter [28]. Within the first hour, hyperventilation reduces $P^*_{CO_2}$ from 160 to less than 80 Torr before intense thermogenesis begins. Lactic acid production is responsible for only half of the metabolic acidosis.

Intracellular acid-base state

In most cells (with the exception of red blood cells), H^+ ions are not passively distributed across the cell membrane according to the membrane potential and the extracellular pH. Instead, intracellular (cytosolic) pH, pHi, is maintained at a nearly constant level above equilibrium by the so-called proton pumps, which actively extrude acidic equivalents across the cell membrane. These 'pumps' are in fact ionic exchange mechanisms, exchanging, for example, Na^+ against protons or Cl^- against bicarbonate ions. When a cell is exposed to an acid load as in a hypercapnia, the efflux of acidic equivalents is increased, thus progressively restoring pHi by metabolic compensation [46]. Except for the short term, intracellular pH is therefore not passively determined by extracellular pH and P_{CO_2}.

Intracellular pH has been determined in tissues of hibernating and aroused hamsters, in winter, using the distribution of a radioactive tracer, the weak acid DMO (dimethyl-oxazolidine, dione) [47]. In this experiment, hibernation blood acid-base state represents a pure respiratory acidosis (Fig. 9). At the intracellular level, a broad distinction can be made between two groups of tissues [23, 48]. In striated muscles and in brain, no significant deviation from the tissue buffer line can be seen, i.e. no clearcut metabolic compensation (or aggravation) of the

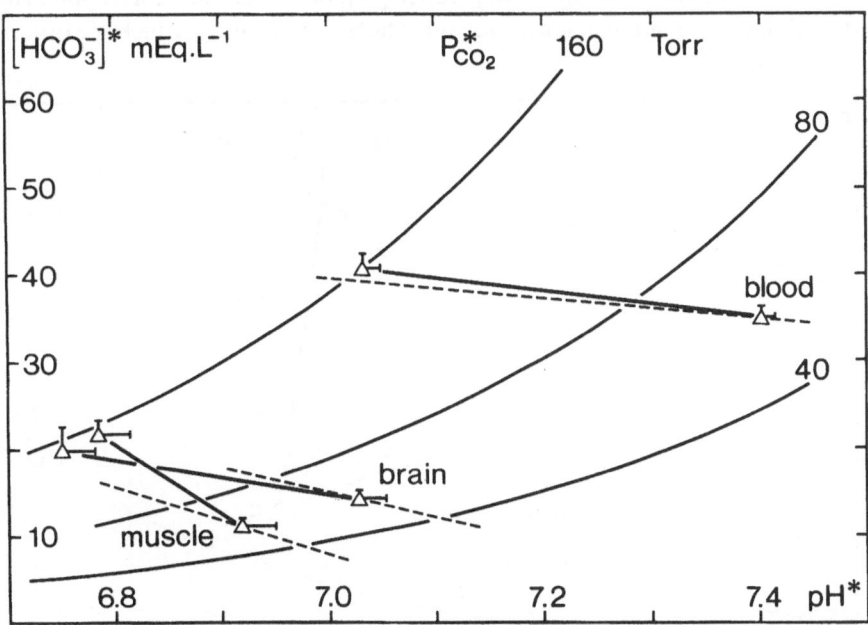

Fig. 9. Temperature-corrected acid-base data of intracellular fluid of skeletal muscle and brain (DMO method), and of (venous) blood plasma in European hamsters, hibernating ($P^*_{CO_2}$ about 160 Torr) or normothermic. Standard temperature is 37° C. Hibernation body temperature was about 10° C. Broken lines are the corresponding buffer lines with slopes of 40, 30 and 11.4 mEq.l^{-1}.pH unit^{-1} respectively. Like blood, intracellular fluid is acidotic in these tissues.

respiratory acidosis takes place. Consequently, pH* and alpha decrease. By contrast, metabolic compensation ensures a near constancy of pHi* - and thereby of alpha - in the liver, and to a lesser extent in the heart (Fig. 10), at the expense of a considerable increase in bicarbonate concentration. This compensation probably results from the accelerated operation of membrane acid-extruding pumps. This is an energy-requiring process, and its occurrence in an otherwise thrifty animal is quite remarkable. Cyclic AMP-mediated hormones facilitate intracellular pH regulation [49] and might intervene here.

Taking into account the respective contributions of the tissues to total body water, in which muscles represent the largest share, the major part of intracellular fluids is acidotic in hibernation. The apparent inhibition of the mechanisms regulating intracellular pH is quite surprising, particularly in brain in which they are the most powerful in normothermy [50]. Of course, the DMO method gives an average over the whole brain, and these results do not preclude the possibility of a local pHi regulation in some restricted brain areas; but if so, pHi would have to be still lower in the rest of the brain to get the same mean value.

Extruding acidic equivalents from the cells to control intracellular pH generates a metabolic acid load in the extracellular compartment. Since extracellular water space is less than half the intracellular water space, an average increase of 1 mEq/l of intracellular strong ion difference [51], or buffer base corresponds to an extracellular acid load of at least 2 mEq/l. The mechanisms by which the organism

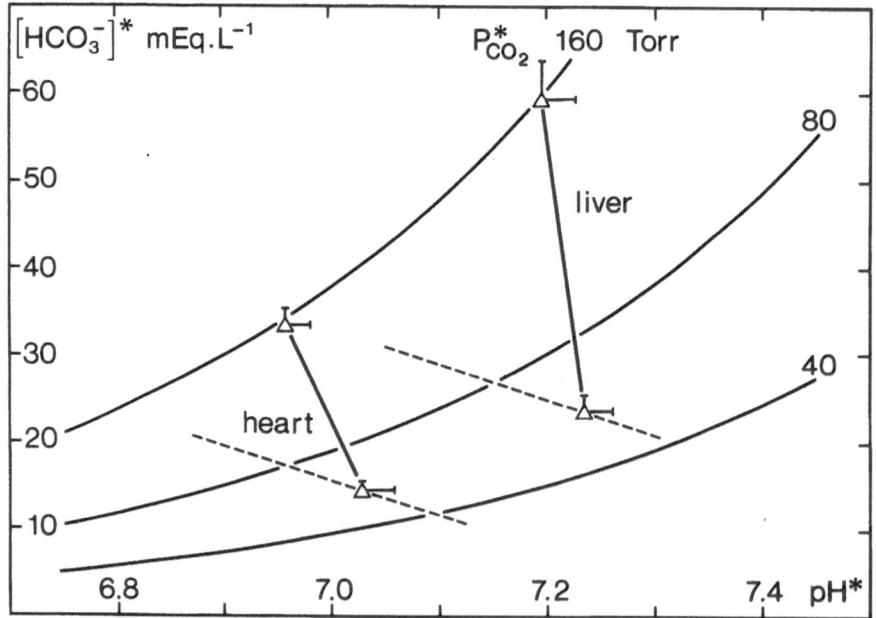

Fig. 10. Same as Fig. 9 for heart and liver. In hibernation, intracellular metabolic compensation tends to bring pH* back to the normothermic value.

keeps the total net flux of acidic equivalents from the cells to the extracellular fluid below the net urinary acid excretion rate are still largely unknown. They may be particularly important in hibernation, since urine production is markedly reduced (there is no voiding of urine).

The acidic equivalents excreted from the heart and liver might be temporarily taken up by bone. Osteoporosis occurs in hibernation in jaw alveolar bone of European hamsters and thirteen-lined ground squirrels [52, 53], in dental bone of ground squirrels [54] and in skull, femur and tibia of hamsters [52]. It was not observed in hind limb bones of ground squirrels [55] and golden hamsters [56], but this may represent a difference between species or bone types.

Inhibition by acidosis

It has been proposed [3, 28, 57, 58] that the respiratory acidosis of hibernation could exert an inhibition on energy utilization and on thermoregulatory mechanisms. As the potential agent of this inhibition, CO_2 has the advantage of being rapidly distributed throughout the body and removed if necessary.

Acidosis affects a variety of cellular processes [reviews in 46, 49, 60]. For instance, intracellular pH is a potent modulator of glycolysis in the red blood cell [61], and in the skeletal muscle in which it mediates the action of insulin [62]. The main site of action of pH is on phosphofructokinase (PFK), a rate-limiting enzyme (Fig. 11) [21]. The activity vs. pH curve is shifted to the right when temperature is decreased, as expected from an imidazole-dependent phenomenon. The normothermic pHi of the hibernator's skeletal muscle in vivo corresponds to the maximal activity of the enzyme. By keeping a nearly constant nominal pHi when going from 37 to 6° C (with a corresponding decrease in pH*), a quite effective inhibition of PFK - and presumably of glycolysis - is achieved in hibernation in the muscle (Fig. 11). By contrast, maintaining nearly constant pH* and alpha in the liver restricts the inhibition to less than 40%.

Similarly, respiratory acidosis strongly inhibits norepinephrine-mediated non-shivering thermogenesis, whose main effector in small mammals is the brown adipose tissue [63]. Compared to the normal $P^*_{CO_2}$, a $P^*_{CO_2}$ of 160 Torr reduces by 50 to 75% the increase in oxygen consumption elicited in isolated brown adipocytes by physiological doses of norepinephrine. Lowering $P^*_{CO_2}$ from 160 to 80 Torr suffices to suppress this inhibition nearly completely at temperatures up to 25° C (Malan, unpubl.). Acidosis also inhibits other effects of norepinephrine, such as its lipolytic action [64].

In normothermic hibernators, hypercapnia depresses the firing rate of temperature sensitive or insensitive neurones of the preoptic area of the hypothalamus, an area involved in temperature detection and regulation [65]. A similar effect may be responsible for the lowering by hypercapnia of the body temperature threshold for shivering (Fig. 12) [66]. In this way, respiratory acidosis

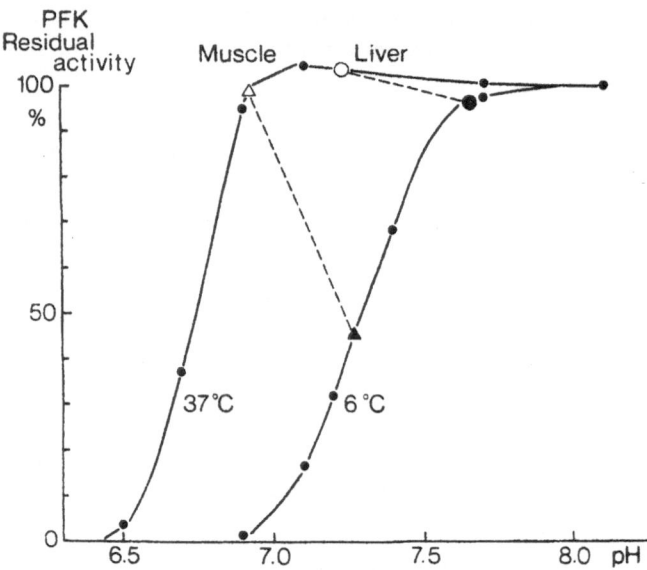

Fig. 11. Effect of pH on the activity of phosphofructokinase from the skeletal muscle of a hibernating mammal (ground squirrel) at 37 and 6° C. Lowering temperature shifts the curve to the right like imidazole pK'. Hamster muscle and liver intracellular pH (same data as Figs. 9 and 10, here not temperature-corrected) are indicated; H, hibernation; N, normothermy. PFK activity is about 55% inhibited in the muscle in hibernation. Inhibition is negligible in the liver owing to the metabolic regulation of pH. Adapted from Hand and Somero [21].

probably intervenes in the downward shift of the regulated body temperature observed in hibernation (Fig. 2).

By accumulating CO_2 in his blood and tissues on entering into torpor, the hibernator thus probably achieves a reversible inhibition of various nervous and metabolic processes, which contributes to the lowering of body temperature and to the sparing of energy reserves. Conversely, the hyperventilation characteristic of early arousal will rapidly bring $P^*_{CO_2}$ back to below 80 Torr, thus returning blood and tissue pH closer to constant alpha conditions. That this takes place before any susbstantial increase in heat production strongly suggests that alpha conservation is required for optimal metabolic efficiency at a low body temperature even in a hibernating mammal.

But the acidosis of hibernation (the 'constant pH' strategy) also has its potential drawbacks. In the perfused rabbit heart at 37° C, left ventricular contractility is reduced 50% by a decrease of pHi of only 0.1 [67]. This may explain why the respiratory acidosis is compensated in the heart by ionic regulation. Similarly in the liver, the delicate balance between the various metabolic pathways characteristic of a starving animal like the hibernator may necessitate a constant alpha, and therefore the observed doubling of bicarbonate concentration to compensate

Spinal temperature

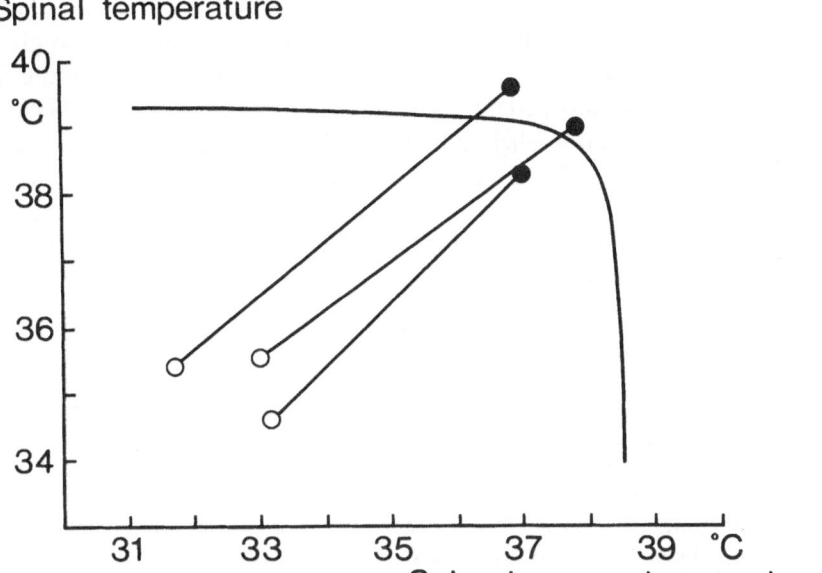

Fig. 12. Shift of threshold temperatures for shivering in guinea pigs during acute exposure to 15% CO_2 (generating a respiratory acidosis less pronounced than in hibernation) (open circles) compared to normocapnic controls (closed circles). In normocapnia, the threshold is a function of both central and peripheral temperatures (solid line). The threshold is lowered for both signals by hypercapnia. Redrawn from Schaefer and Wünnenberg [66].

the respiratory acidosis. A powerfull - and probably costly - intracellular alpha regulation in two organs essential for survival, heart and liver, probably represents the price the hibernator has to pay to make use of the inhibition by acidosis.

Conclusion: Is the hibernation model applicable to human patients?

The experimental studies on hibernation do not justify the earlier claims that mammals differ from other vertebrates with respect to pH-temperature relationships. For mammalian tissues, as for amphibian or reptilian tissues, alphastat regulation represents the normal, or neutral, acid-base condition when temperature is varied. This is supported by in vitro studies of blood and enzymes of active heterothermic mammals, and by the observations of blood pH* regulation during arousal, and of intracellular pH* regulation in heart and liver in hibernation.

In spite of the constancy of nominal, or temperature-uncorrected pH, the acid-base state during hibernation results from the combined effects of low temperature and a severe respiratory acidosis. This acidosis probably contributes to the inhibition of various metabolic and nervous processes observed in hibernation. Although such inhibitory effects might seem to be useful in certain clinical situations, exposing humans to an acute acidosis (the 'constant pH' strategy) may not be without risks, especially for heart function. It may also fail to give the expected results: artificial hypercapnia does not inhibit nonshivering thermogenesis like the self-imposed hypercapnia of hibernation, probably because of the catecholamine secretion elicited by forced hypercapnia [65]. And we ignore the mechanisms by which the hibernator can selectively facilitate intracellular pH regulation in the heart and liver to prevent adverse effects of acidosis, while inhibiting it in most of the organism including the brain.

References

1. Lyman CP: Who is who among the hibernators. In: Hibernation and Torpor in Mammals and Birds, Lyman CP, Willis JS, Malan A, Wang, LCH. Academic Press, New York, 1982: 12–36.
2. Kayser C: La dépense d'énergie des mammifères en hibernation. Arch Sci Physiol 18: 137–150, 1964.
3. Malan A: Enzyme regulation, metabolic rate and acid-base state in hibernation. In: Animals and Environmental Fitness, Gilles R (ed). Pergamon Press, Oxford, 1980: 487–501.
4. Kayser C: The Physiology of Natural Hibernation. Pergamon Press, Oxford, 1961.
5. Wang LCH: Energetic and field aspects of mammalian torpor: The Richardson's ground squirrel. In: Strategies in Cold: Natural Torpidity and Thermogenesis, Wang LC, Hudson JW (eds). Academic Press, New York, 1978: 109–145.
6. Heler HC, Colliver GW: CNS regulation of body temperature during hibernation. Am J Physiol 227: 583–589, 1974.
7. Heller HC, Colliver GW, Anand P: CNS regulation of body temperature in euthermic hibernators. Am J Physiol 227: 576–582, 1974.
8. Heller HC, Colliver GW, Beard J: Thermoregulation during entrance into hibernation. Pflügers Arch 369: 55–59, 1977.
9. Heller HC, Walker GM, Florant GL, Glotzbach SF, Berger RJ: Sleep and hibernation: Electrophysiological and thermoregulatory homologies. In: Strategies in Cold: Natural Torpidity and Thermogenesis, Wang LC, Hudson JW (eds). Academic Press, New York, 1978: 225–265.
10. Chatfield PO, Lyman CP: Subcortical electrical activity in the golden hamster during arousal from hibernation. Electroencephalogr Clin Neurophysiol 6: 403–408, 1954.
11. Kayser C, Malan A: Central nervous system and hibernation. Experientia 19: 1–11, 1963.
12. Kilduff TS, Sharp FR, Heller HC: [14C] 2-deoxyglucose uptake in ground squirrel brain during hibernation. J Neuroscience 2: 143–157, 1982.
13. Lyman CP: Sensitivity to arousal. In: Hibernation and Torpor in Mammals and Birds, Lyman CP, Willis JS, Malan A, Wang LCH. Academic Press, New York, 1982: 77–91.
14. Behrisch HW: Metabolic economy at the biochemical level: The hibernator. In: Strategies in Cold: Natural Torpidity and Thermogenesis, Wang LCH, Hudson JW (eds). Academic Press, New York, 1978: 461–497.
15. Behrisch HW, Smullin DH, Morse GA: Life at low and changing temperatures. In: Survival in the Cold. Musacchia XJ, Jansky L (eds). Elsevier-North Holland, New York, 1981: 191–212.
16. Borgmann AI, Moon TW: Enzymes of the normothermic and hibernating bat. *Myotis lucifugus:* temperature as a modulator of pyruvate kinase. J Comp Physiol 107B: 185–199, 1976.
17. Charnock JS: Membrane lipid phase-transitions: a possible biological response to hibernation? In: Strategies in Cold: Natural Torpidity and Thermogenesis, Wang LCH, Hudson JW (eds). Academic Press, New York, 1978: 417–460.
18. Malan A: Adaptation to poikilothermy in endotherms. J Therm Biol 8: 79–84, 1983.

19. Moon TW, Borgmann AI: Enzymes of the normothermic and hibernating bat, *Myotis lucifugus:* metabolites as modulators of pyruvate kinase. J Comp Physiol 107B: 201–210, 1976.
20. Behrisch HW, Ortner I, Wieser W: Temperature and regulation of enzyme activity in heterothermic tissues of an alpine mammal. Lactate dehydrogenase from skeletal muscle of the chamois. J Therm Biol 2: 185–189, 1977.
21. Hand SC, Somero GN: Phosphofructokinase of the hibernator *Citellus beecheyi*: Temperature and pH regulation of activity via influences on the tetramer-dimer equilibrium. Physiol Zool 56: 380–388, 1983.
22. Templeton JR: Reptiles. In: Comparative Physiology of Thermoregulation, Vol. 1. Whittow GC (ed). Academic Press, New York, 1970: 167–221.
23. Malan A: Respiration and acid-base state in hibernation. In: Hibernation and Torpor in Mammals and Birds, Lyman CP, Willis JS, Malan A, Wang LCH. Academic Press, New York, 1982: 237–282.
24. Grande F: Man under caloric deficiency. In: Handbook of Physiology. Sect. 4: Adaptation t) the Environment, Dill DB (ed). Am Physiol Soc, Washington, D.C.: 911–937.
25. Le Maho Y: Metabolic adaptations to long-term fasting in antarctic penguins and domestic geese. J Therm Biol 8: 91–96, 1983.
26. Lyman CP: Effect of increased CO_2 on respiration and heart rate of hibernating hamsters and ground squirrels. Am J Physiol 167: 638–643, 1951.
27. Tähti H: Effects of changes in CO_2 and O_2 concentrations in the inspired gas on respiration in the hibernating hedgehog *(Erinaceus europaeus L.)* Ann Zool Fenn 12: 183–187, 1975.
28. Malan A, Arens H, Waechter A: Pulmonary respiration and acid-base state in hibernating marmots and hamsters. Respir Physiol 17: 45–61, 1973.
29. Bickler PE: Blood acid-base status of an awake heterothermic rodent, *Spermophilus tereticaudus*. Respir Physiol 57: 307–316.
30. Rodeau JL: The effect of temperature on intracellular pH in crayfish neurones and muscle fibers. Am J Physiol 246: C45–C49, 1984.
31. Walsh PJ, Moon TW: Intracellular pH-temperature interactions of hepatocytes from American eels. Am J Physiol 245: R32–R37, 1983.
32. Hitzig BM: Temperature-induced changes in turtle CSF pH and central control of ventilation. Resp Physiol 49: 205–222, 1982.
33. Reeves RB: Temperature induced changes in blood acid-base status: pH and P_{CO_2} in a binary buffer. J Appl Physiol 40: 752–761, 1976.
34. Reeves RB: Temperature induced changes in blood acid-base status: Donnan r_{Cl} and red cell volume. J Appl Physiol 40: 762–767, 1976.
35. Reeves RB: An imidazole alphastat hypothesis for vertebrate acid-base regulation: tissue carbon dioxide content and body temperature in bullfrogs. Respir Physiol 14: 219–236, 1972.
36. Malan A: Blood acid-base state at a variable temperature. A graphical representation. Respir Physiol 31: 259–275, 1977.
37. Rodeau JL, Malan A: A two compartment model of blood acid-base state state at constant or variable temperature. Respir Physiol 37: 5–30.
38. Funder J, Wieth JO: Chloride and hydrogen ion distribution between human red cells and plasma. Acta Physiol Scand 68: 234–245, 1966.
39. Woodbury JW: Regulation of pH. In: Physiology and Biophysics, Ruch TC, Patton HD (eds). Saunders, Philadelphia, Pa., 1965: 899–938.
40. Snapp BD, Heller HC: Suppression of metabolism during hibernation in ground squirrels *(Citellus lateralis)*. Physiol Zool 54: 297–307, 1981.
41. Dontcheff L, Kayser C: Explication de certains quotients respiratoires aberrants chez les hibernants. C.R. Soc. Biol. (Paris) 118: 81–83, 1934.
42. Kayser C, Rietsch ML, Lucot MA: Les échanges respiratoires et la fréquence cardiaque des hibernants au cours du réveil de leur sommeil hivernal. Arch Sci Physiol 8: 155–194, 1954.

52

43. Cannon B, Nedergaard J, Sundin U: Thermogenesis, brown fat and thermogenin. In: Survival in the Cold, Musacchia XJ, Jansky L (eds). Elsevier-North Holland, New York, 1981: 99–120.
44. Lyman CP: Mechanisms of arousal. In: Hibernation and Torpor in Mammals and Birds, Lyman CP, Willis JS, Malan A, Wang LCH. Academic Press, New York 1982: 104–123.
45. Lyman CP: The oxygen consumption and temperature regulation of hibernating hamsters. J Exp Zool 109: 55–78, 1948.
46. Roos A, Boron WF: Intracellular pH. Physiol Rev 61: 296–434, 1981.
47. Poole DT, Butler TC, Waddell WJ: Intracellular pH of the Ehrlich ascites tumor cell. J Natl Cancer Inst 32: 939–946, 1964.
48. Malan A, Rodeau JL, Daull R: Intracellular pH in hibernating hamsters. Cryobiology 18: 100–101, 1981.
49. Fenton RA, Gonzalez NC, Clancy RL: The effect of dibutyryl cyclic AMP and glucagon on the myocardial cell pH. Respir Physiol 32: 213–223, 1978.
50. Messeter K, Siesjö BK: The intracellular pH' in the brain in acute and sustained hypercapnia. Acta Physiol Scand 83: 210–219, 1971.
51. Stewart PA: Independent and dependent variables of acid-base control. Respir Physiol 33: 9–26, 1978.
52. Kayser C, Franck RM: Comportement des tissus calcifiés du hamster d'Europe Cricetus cricetus au cours de l'hibernation. Arch Oral Biol 8: 703–718, 1963.
53. Haller AC, Zimny ML: Effects of hibernation on interradicular alveolar bone. J Dent Res 56: 1552–1557, 1977.
54. Zimny ML, Haller AC: Effects of hibernation on dental tissues: a SEM analytical study. Comp Biochem Physiol 60A, 257–262, 1978.
55. Zimmerman GD, McKean TA, Hardt AB: Hibernation and disuse osteoporosis. Cryobiology 13: 84–94, 1976.
56. Tempel GE, Wolinsky I, Musacchia XJ: Bone and serum calcium in normothermic, cold-acclimated and hibernating hamsters. Comp Biochem Physiol 61A: 145–147, 1978.
57. Dubois R: Etude sur le mécanisme de la thermogenèse et du sommeil chez les mammifères. Physiologie comparée de la marmotte. Ann Univ Lyon 25, 1896.
58. Malan A: Hibernation as a model for studies on thermogenesis and its control. In: Effectors of Thermogenesis, Girardier L, Seydoux J (eds). Birkhäuser, Basel, 1978: 303–314.
59. Cohen RD, Isles RA: Intracellular pH: measurement, control and metabolic interrelationships. CRC Crit Rev Clin Lab Sci 6: 101–143, 1975.
60. Nuccitelli R, Deamer DW: Intracellular pH: Its Measurement, Regulation, and Utilization in Cellular Functions. Alan R. Liss, New York, 1982.
61. Tomoda A, Tsuda-Hirota S, Minakami S: Glycolysis of red cells suspended in solutions of impermeable solutes. Intracellular pH and glycolysis. J Biochem (Tokyo) 81: 697–701, 1977.
62. Fidelman ML, Seeholzer KB, Walsh KB, Moore RD: Intracellular pH mediates action of insulin on glycolysis in frog skeletal muscle. Am J Physiol 242: C87–C93, 1982.
63. Pepelko WE, Dixon GA: Elimination of cold-induced nonshivering thermogenesis by hypercapnia. Am J Physiol 227: 264–267, 1974.
64. Nahas GC, Poyart C: Effect of arterial pH alterations on metabolic activity of norepinephrine. Am J Physiol 212: 765–772, 1967.
65. Wünnenberg W, Baltruschat D: Temperature regulation of golden hamsters during acute hypercapnia. J Therm Biol 7: 83–86, 1982.
66. Schaefer KE, Wünnenberg W: Threshold temperatures for shivering in acute and chronic hypercapnia. J Appl Physiol 41: 67–70, 1976.
67. Jacobus WE, Pores IH, Lucas SK, Kallman CH, Weisfeldt ML, Flaherty JT: The role of intracellular pH in the control of normal and ischemic myocardial contractility: A ^{31}P nuclear magnetic resonance and mass spectrometry study. In: Intracellular pH: Its Measurement, Regulation and Utilization in Cellular Functions, Nuccitelli R, Deamer DW (eds). Alan R. Liss, New York, 1982: 537–565.

68. Clausen G: Acid-base balance in the hedgehog *Erinaceus europaeus (L.)* during hibernation hypothermia, cooling and rewarming. Arbok Univ Bergen, Mat.-Naturvitensk Ser No. 6: 1–11, 1966.
69. Tähti H, Soivio A: Blood gas concentrations, acid-base balance and blood pressure in hedgehogs in the active state and in hibernation with periodic respiration. Ann Zool Fenn 12: 188–192, 1975.
70. Kent KM, Peirce EC,II: Acid-base characteristics of hibernating animals. J Appl Physiol 23: 336–340, 1967.
71. Musacchia XJ, Volkert WA: Blood gases in hibernating and active ground squirrels: HbO_2 affinity at 6 and 38°C. Am J Physiol 221: 128–130, 1971.
72. Goodrich CA: Acid-base balance in euthermic and hibernating marmots. Am J Physiol 224: 1185–1189, 1973.
73. Kreienbühl G, Strittmatter J, Ayim E: Blood gas analyses of hibernating hamsters and dormice Pflügers Arch 336: 167–172, 1976.
74. Bickler PE: CO_2 balance of a heterothermic rodent: comparison of sleep, torpor, and awake states. Am J Physiol 246: R49–R55.

4. Enzymatic consequences under alphastat regulation

GEORGE N. SOMERO and FRED N. WHITE

Abstract

The importance of conserving the fractional protonation state of histidyl imidazole groups (alphastat pH regulation) is discussed for key structural and functional properties of proteins. For enzymes like lactate dehydrogenase (LDH) which have active site histidyl residues involved in the binding and catalytic events, the advantages of alphastat regulation are seen in the conservation of binding ability (as estimated by apparent Michaelis constants), of catalytic reserve capacity (the ability to respond effectively to changes in substrate concentration) and of reaction reversibility. For enzymes which depend on histidyl residues for their integrity of subunit assembly, e.g., phosphofructokinase (PFK), alphastat regulation ensures the maintenance of the active, assembled structure under different temperatures, and the regulatory responsiveness of the protein is also conserved. These advantages to enzymes of alphastat regulation during changes in body temperature are seen both in short-term changes in body temperature and in evolutionary adaptation to temperature.

From the observed effects of changes in temperature and pH on enzyme systems studied in vitro, predictions are made about the effects of alphastat and pHstat (constant pH at all temperatures) regimens on more complex, physiological systems. These predictions, e.g., of alphastat and pHstat effects on total glycolytic flux and partitioning of glucose carbon between lactate and pyruvate, are compared with existing data from studies of whole organisms or isolated, perfused organs. The predictions from enzymatic studies are largely supported, and the critical importance of alphastat regulation in the maintenance of organ function under hypothermic conditions is apparent.

The benefits of alphastat regulation are also discussed in the contexts of maintaining pH gradients across the inner mitochondrial membrane, of keeping the activities of pH-sensitive enzymes near optimal pH values, and of maintaining maximal buffering capacities. Lastly, the activation of several physiological systems by eliminating an acidotic state and restoring an alphastat pH value is presented to show the widespread significance, in both natural and clinical settings, of alphastat regulation for metabolic function.

Introduction

Analyses by Rahn and Reeves and their colleagues [1–5] of pH relationships in both mammalian and ecothermic ('cold-blooded') animals illustrate especially well one of the major contributions that the comparative approach to physiology and biochemistry can make. Through comparative study of the way in which widely different animals cope with a comman problem, and of the so-called 'solutions' attained by these different animals to resolve this problem, we often can obtain an unequaled perspective of the fundamental objectives of physiological and biochemical regulation. In the case at hand, that of alphastat regulation of intracellular pH (pH_i), the observation that most tissues of nearly all animals (with some interesting exceptions we treat later) regulate pH_i so as to conserve the protonation state (alpha-imidazole) of histidine imidazole groups at all temperatures offers a compelling reason for viewing the degree of imidazole protonation as an especially critical feature of the cell's biochemistry. In this essay we discuss the reasons why imidazole protonation is so important for a variety of enzymatic functions, and why the failure of pH_i to approximate the pK of the imidazole group (pK_{imid}) can have serious consequences for a broad spectrum of physiological activities. We will give special attention to interactions between body temperature and pH_i. As Reeves' analysis in this volume has clearly shown, to maintain an appropriate intracellular milieu for protein function in the face of changing body temperature, pH_i must be regulated such that a rise in pH_i of approximately 0.017 pH unit occurs for each degree Celsius fall in body temperature. That is, pH_i must change with temperature in parallel with pK_{imid}. These relationships, which are discussed more fully by Reeves in chapter 2 are portrayed in Fig. 1.

To appreciate the physiological significance of alphastat pH regulation, i.e., of the conservation of imidazole protonation state, we will examine the effects of imidazole protonation state on the catalytic and structural properties of enzymes for which histidine residues serve as key features of the catalytic mechanism and the maintenance of enzyme structure. We also will examine cases in which alphastat regulation may preserve metabolic function even when histidine imidazole protonation effects may not be key elements in the metabolic system. The conclusions we draw, and the predictions we make, from the results of these in vitro studies of isolated enzymes will then be compared to data obtained from studies in which metabolic perturbations have been effected through experimental manipulation of in vivo pH_i values.

Lactate dehydrogenase: pH effects on pyruvate and lactate metabolism

An appropriate starting point for our analysis of pH_i effects on enzyme systems is the lactate dehydrogenase (LDH, EC 1.1.1.27) reaction, the terminal reaction of

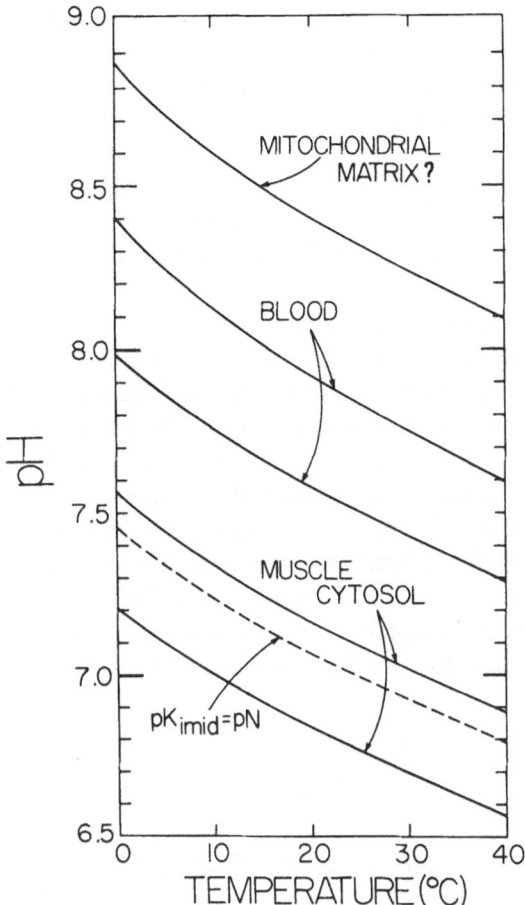

Fig. 1. Relationship of blood, muscle cytosol, and mitochondrial matrix pH to body temperature in ectothermic animals. The effect of temperature on the pK of imidazole (pKi_{mid}) and the neutral pH of water (pN) is shown by the dashed line. The pairs of lines for the blood and muscle cytosol bracket the range of experimentally determined values for the pH's of these fluids in a large number of studies. The line for the pH of mitochondrial matrix is hypothetical since the pH of this compartment has not been measured as a function of temperature, but is probably 1 to 1.5 pH units more alkaline than the pH of the cytosol. The figure is modified after [9].

the glycolytic sequence. LDH plays a critical role in glycogen and glucose metabolism by regenerating oxidized cofactor (NAD^+) to sustain glycolytic function under conditions of limiting oxygen. Thus, when functioning in the pyruvate reductase mode, LDH catalyzes the reaction:

$$\text{pyruvate} + \text{NADH} + \text{H}^+ \rightleftharpoons \text{lactate} + \text{NAD}^+.$$

This often is the direction of LDH function in skeletal muscle tissue, in which the demands for ATP generation during intense locomotor activity cannot be met entirely by oxidative reactions of the electron transport system, due to limitations

58

in oxygen delivery to the tissues and mitochondria. In aerobically-poised tissues like heart, LDH typically functions as a lactate oxidase system, converting lactate to pyruvate. The latter metabolite subsequently can be directed into the Krebs citric acid cycle after being converted into the two-carbon unit, acetylCoA, by the pyruvate dehydrogenase reaction. We see, therefore, that LDH must play different roles in different tissues, and under different physiological conditions, for example, oxygen supply. How are these roles fulfilled, and what are the consequences of changes in pH_i and body temperature (T_B) on the rate and the direction of LDH function?

To approach these questions it is essential to examine first the role played by histidine imidazole groups in LDH function. Figure 2 illustrates in a simplified manner the structure of the active site of LDH, and the types of interactions that occur between the substrate (pyruvate is shown), the cofactor (NADH), and the amino acid residues of the active site. Pyruvate is anchored to the active site by two principal types of interactions, those with arginine-171 (ARG-171) and those with histidine-195 (HIS-195). An important difference between the pyruvate-ARG and pyruvate-HIS interactions is that ARG-171 will always have a positive charge at physiological pH values, while HIS-195 imidazole groups, under alpha-stat conditions, where pH_i is apt to be slightly below pK_{imid} (see Fig. 1), will be just over half in the protonated state. Since pyruvate is able to bind to the LDH active

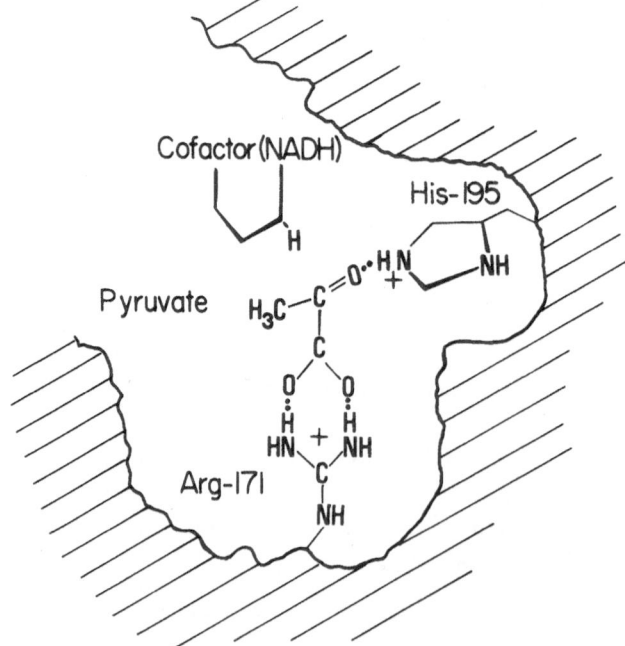

Fig. 2. Simplified representation of the active site of lactate dehydrogenase, illustrating the roles played by ARG-171 and HIS-195 in stabilizing enzyme-substrate binding. Shown is pyruvate, which binds only to the protonated form of the imidazole ring of HIS-195.

site only when HIS-195 is protonated, it follows that small changes in pH$_i$ can lead to substantial shifts in the ability of LDH to bind pyruvate. This relationship is shown in Fig. 3, which portrays the effect of changes in pH$_i$ on the reaction rate of an enzyme system in which, as in the case of LDH, substrate binding is enhanced by falling pH. As shown in this figure, the ability of slight changes in pH$_i$ to affect the rate of the reaction depends upon substrate concentrations being less than saturating; pH has no effect on the maximal velocity (V$_{max}$) of the LDH reaction. In fact, within cells the concentrations of substrates for most enzymes are maintained near or below the value of the apparent Michaelis constant (K$_m$) of substrate, the concentration of substrate yielding one-half V$_{max}$ [6, 7]. For most enzymatic reactions, then, physiological substrate concentrations permit only about one-half or less of the potential rate of the reaction found under saturating concentrations of substrate. As discussed later, for the skeletal muscle isozyme of LDH (the 'muscle-type' or 'M$_4$' isozyme) the K$_m$ of pyruvate for LDH homologues of a wide variety of vertebrates, including fishes, reptiles, birds, and mammals, lies in the range of 0.15 to 0.35 mM pyruvate, at physiological temperatures and pH [7–10]. Concentrations of pyruvate in resting skeletal muscle of different vertebrates range between 0.01 and 0.30 mmol/kg fresh weight of tissue [7, 8, 11]. Thus, at least under conditions of minimal locomotory activity, the LDH system of vertebrate skeletal muscle typically functions well below its V$_{max}$ potential.

At first glance it may seem paradoxical that many enzymes are exposed to

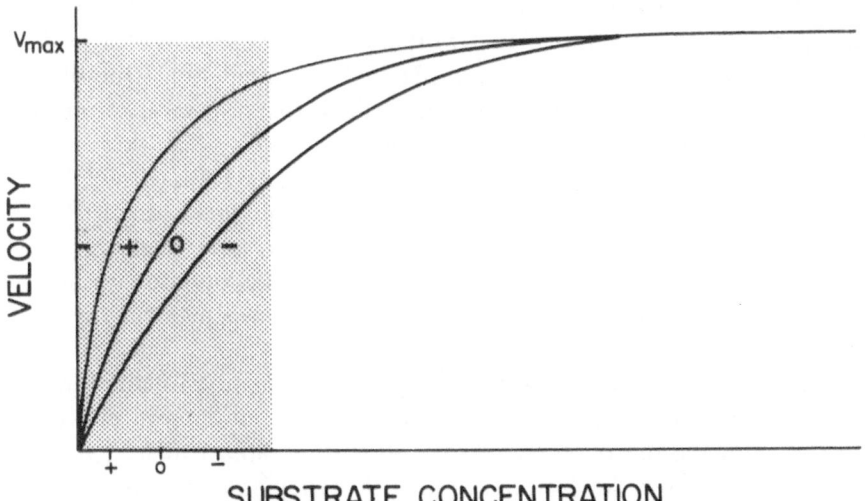

Fig. 3. Effects of changes in pH on the activity of an enzyme which, like LDH (see Fig. 2), has a pH-dependent affinity for substrate due to the occurrence of a binding interaction between substrate and an imidazole ring. The curve labeled 'O' represents an intracellular pH value lying near the alphastat value (pH$_i$ near to or slightly below pK$_{imid}$; see Fig. 1). Curves labeled '+' and '−' portray the effects of increases and decreases in proton activity, respectively. The symbols on the abscissa denote the K$_m$ of substrate at these three different pH values. Stippling indicates the range of intracellular substrate, e.g., pyruvate, concentrations.

substrate concentrations in vivo that are able to support rates of catalysis that are only a fraction of V_{max}. However, enzymes must not only be powerful catalysts that are able to drive metabolism at high rates, but they also must be sensitive regulators of metabolic rates. In this latter role as regulatory elements, enzymes extract great benefit from the non-saturating substrate concentrations present in their milieu. For the LDH reaction functioning in the pyruvate reductase mode, the fact that pyruvate concentrations in resting muscle are generally below K_m levels means that, during vigorous exercise when the breakdown of glycogen is accelerated, the LDH reaction can respond to increases in pyruvate production (concentration) with rapid, large-scale increases in pyruvate reductase activity. That is, the subsaturating relationships between enzymes and their substrates ensure that a critical reserve capacity exists in metabolic pathways.

Returning now to the significance of alphastat regulation for LDH function, we can appreciate that the fall in pH_i of muscle that accompanies anaerobic glycolysis can have an important regulatory effect on LDH function. Protons generated during lactate production will titrate the imidazole group of HIS-195, and thereby lower the K_m of pyruvate (increase pyruvate binding ability). Alphastat regulation maintains imidazole titration curves in their steepest regions, so even slight changes in pH_i can be translated into large changes in enzymatic activity. For LDH, slight decreases in pH_i of the muscle cytosol, therefore, can increase the activity of an enzyme whose function is critical for sustained glycolytic activity under oxygen-limiting conditions.

It is pertinent to note in this context that a common feature of hypothermic patients under conditions of constant pH (pHstat) regulation (true blood pH maintained at 7.4) is lactic acidosis. Here, it is likely that protons generated by the imposed respiratory acidosis may be responsible for this effect by favoring the pyruvate reductase (= lactate generating) activity of LDH. Blayo et al. [12] have shown that for hypothermic patients undergoing cardiac bypass surgery, $[HCO^-_3]$ is maintained under alphastat conditions, and that no lactic acidosis occurs. It thus seems likely that blood pH of 7.4 under hypothermic conditions creates lactic acidosis even in the presence of ample supplies of oxygen to support aerobic metabolism.

A second important consequence of alphastat regulation for the function of enzymes having histidines involved in the catalytic mechanism concerns the reversibility of the reaction. The preservation of an approximately half-protonated state of active site histidine imidazole groups allows a reversibility of function that is critical for many enzymes, including LDH. As discussed earlier, when activation of locomotor muscle function dictates a need for enhanced pyruvate reductase activity by LDH, slight decreases in pH_i can achieve this result. Upon cessation of locomotory activity, the concomitant increase in pH_i will also have an appropriate effect on LDH activity. Under conditions of rising pH_i the ability to bind pyruvate decreases and the affinity for lactate increases. Lactate can bind only to the deprotonated imidazole group of HIS-195 (see Fig.

2). The physiological significance of this change in lactate binding ability should be obvious. Thus, once metabolism of the muscle returns to an aerobic poise, it is appropriate to burn lactate, rather than to form it from pyruvate. The back-titration of HIS-195 by rising pH_i has effect of shifting the preferred direction of LDH function from pyruvate reductase activity to lactate oxidation.

To summarize our analysis of the significance of alphastat regulation for the function of LDH and other enzymes having histidine residues as key contributors to binding and/or catalysis, it is sufficient to reiterate the following points. First, alphastat regulation, by maintaining pH_i near pK_{imid}, maintains these enzymes in a state of maximal sensitivity to changes in pH_i. That is, the imidazole groups are poised at the steepest regions of their titration curves. Second, because of this sensitivity to pH_i, protons can serve as effective regulatory signals for altering both the rates and the directions of metabolic flux. And, suffice it to say, when alphastat regulation is not maintained, severe impairment of metabolic rates and of metabolic regulation can occur, as we illustrate later in our review.

LDH-temperature-pH interactions: An evolutionary perspective

Our analysis of the interactions of temperature and pH on the function of lactate dehydrogenases has, up to this point, emphasized the influences of short-term temperature and pH effects on this reaction. To appreciate more fully the biological consequences of alphastat regulation, it behooves us to broaden our focus, and to consider how alphastat regulation can contribute to adaptation of enzyme function over evolutionary time courses. Specifically, we shall inquire in this section whether the conservation of critical enzymatic properties, like K_m values, can be achieved entirely by appropriate adjustments in pH, or whether the conservation of these critical traits is the joint result of changes in amino acid composition of the protein and appropriate physiological regulation of the milieu in which the protein functions.

The M_4-LDHs of vertebrates offer an appropriate study system for addressing the latter question. Homologous variants of the enzyme have been purified from a wide variety of vertebrates, whose body temperatures span a range of approximately 50° C, from −1.86° C for the Antarctic fish, *Pagothenia borchgrevinki*, to 47° C, the upper core temperature recorded for the thermophilic desert iguana, *Dipsosaurus dorsalis*. The influences of temperature on the K_m of pyruvate for a number of M_4-LDHs are shown in Fig. 4. The K_m values all were determined using an alphastat pH regimen, shown in the inset to the figure [8, 10]. The dark segments of the lines connecting the K_m values indicate the body temperature ranges for the different species.

These data show that the K_m of pyruvate is strongly conserved among species, despite the fact that variations in temperature can strongly effect K_m. Addressing the question raised at the beginning of this section, that concerning the roles

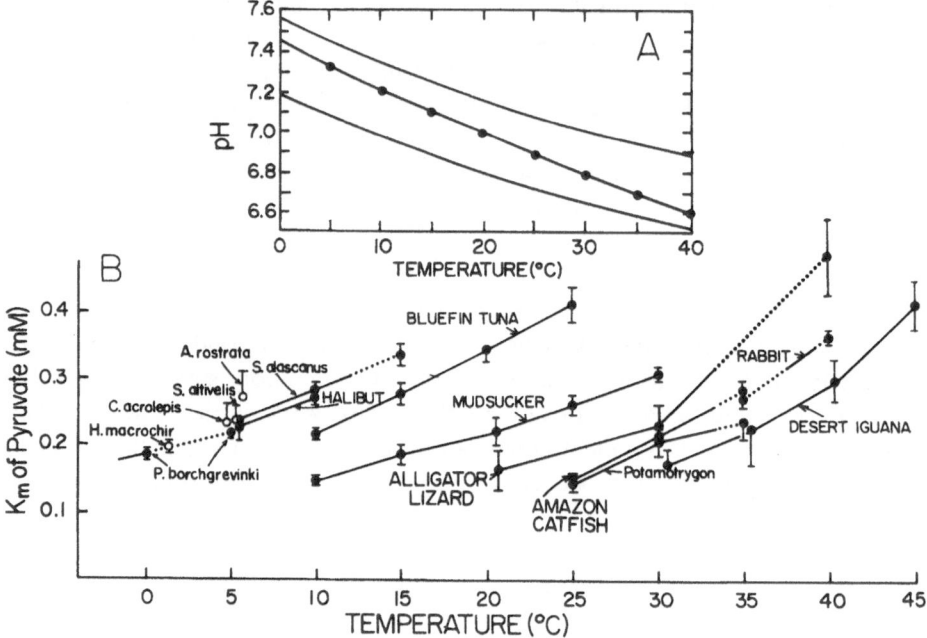

Fig. 4. Frame A. The pH regimen used to determine the K_m values shown in Frame B. The light lines bracket the range of intracellular pH values determined in muscle tissue of a number of vertebrates (see Fig. 1). The darker line connecting the closed symbols indicates the pH of the imidazole/Cl buffer system used in the assays. Frame B. The influence of temperature on the K_m of pyruvate for M_4-LDHs of vertebrates having different body temperatures. The species studied include a mammal (rabbit), two reptiles (the alligator lizard and desert iguana), and a variety of fishes (all other species shown). The open symbols designate deep-sea fishes. The darker regions of the lines connecting the measured K_m values indicate the body temperatures of the species. 95% confidence intervals around the K_m values are shown. The figure is modified after [10].

played by alphastat pH regulation, on the one hand, and evolutionary changes in amino acid composition, on the other hand, in conserving K_m values, we can see that substantial differences exist among the LDH homologs. At any single measurement temperature, the K_m of pyruvate is lowest for the LDHs of the most warm-adapted species, e.g., mammals and desert reptiles. This observation suggests that the conservation of the protonation state of HIS-195 that is achieved by alphastat regulation is not, in and of itself, sufficient to conserve adequately the K_m of pyruvate across all species. In addition to the conservation of K_m that accrues from alphastat pH regulation, amino acid substitutions in the enzymes have been necessary to offset the tendency of increases in temperature to disrupt the binding of pyruvate to the active site. The need for these amino acid substitutions is not surprising in view of the occurrence of additional binding interactions between pyruvate and LDH besides those involving HIS-195 (Fig. 2). Since the interaction between pyruvate and ARG-171, for instance, would also be disrupted by increases in temperature, amino acid substitutions to offset this effect are needed to stabilize the interaction between the enzyme and its substrate in the face of temperature changes.

The complementary roles played by alphastat regulation and amino acid substitutions in conserving K_m values are indicated by the data plotted in Fig. 5. Here the very different responses of K_m to temperature changes noted under alphastat and under pHstat regimens are clearly shown. Under pHstat conditions (phosphate buffer, pH 7.4 at all assay temperatures; see figure legend) the K_m of pyruvate varies approximately 9-fold among the species, and variation in K_m with temperature for each homolog is high. Under alphastat regulation (imidazole buffer with a pH versus temperature relationship like that shown in the inset of Fig. 4), the K_m of pyruvate is much less affected by shifts in assay temperature, and among species the variation in K_m is much less than the variation found under pHstat conditions.

To summarize, alphastat regulation effects a substantial conservation in the K_m of pyruvate in the face of fluctuations in temperature that tend to perturb pyruvate-LDH interactions. The role of alphastat regulation in this conservation

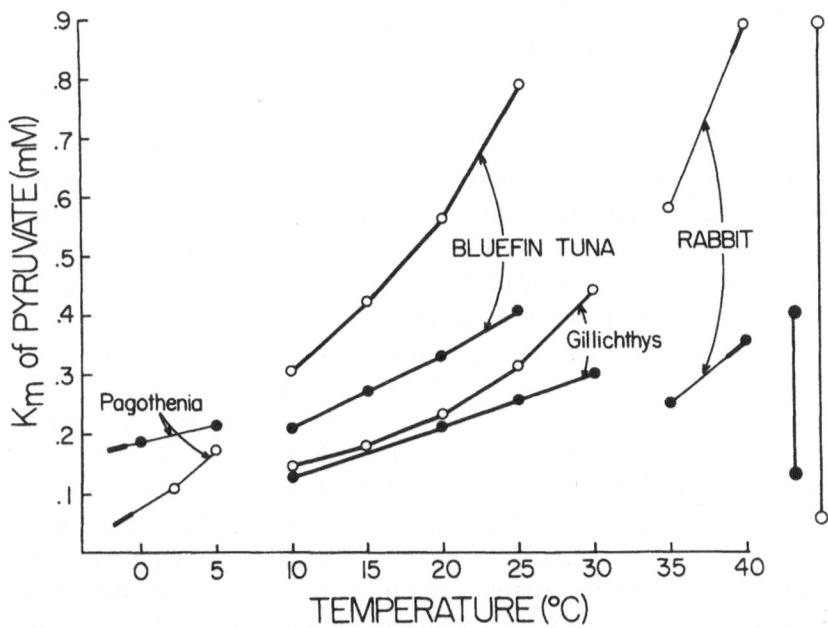

Fig. 5. Effects of experimental temperature on the apparent K_m of pyruvate for vertebrate M_4-LDHs assayed under two different pH regimens: alphastat (closed symbols) and pHstat (open symbols). The alphastat regimen consisted of an 80 mM imidazole/Cl buffer system which had the pH versus temperature response shown in Fig. 4. The pHstat regimen used a 66.7 mM phosphate buffer, pH 7.4 at all measurement temperatures. The vertical lines at the right side of the figure illustrate the ranges of K_m values observed, at physiological temperatures, under the two pH regimens. The species include a mammal (rabbit) and three fishes adapted to different ranges of body temperature (see Fig. 4 for additional examples of the K_m versus temperature response of M_4-LDHs). The figure is modified after [9].

is seen over two very different time courses, those of short-term alterations in body temperature, and evolutionary periods. During evolutionary adaptation to different temperatures, amino acid substitutions occur which complement the K_m stabilizing effects caused by alphastat regulation. Through alphastat pH regulation and these amino acid substitutions, critical enzymatic traits are conserved within fairly narrow limits among animals having widely different body temperatures. We propose that the complementary influences of alphastat regulation and amino acid substitutions found for vertebrate LDHs are quite typical of many protein based processes in which the conservation of a key trait must be maintained over a wide range of temperatures.

Phosphofructokinase: pH and temperature effects on subunit assembly and catalysis

LDH is positioned at the bottom of the glycolytic pathway and directs the flow of carbon between anaerobic and aerobic channels. Positioned near the top of the glycolytic sequence is phosphofructokinase (PFK, EC 2.7.1.11) the enzyme that is primarily responsible for establishing the total flux through glycolysis, whether the pathway is operating under aerobic or anaerobic conditions [13]. In this critical regulatory capacity, PFK must be highly responsive to a broad suite of metabolite signals that indicate the cell's and the organism's needs for glycolytic ATP generation. PFK is activated by falling ATP concentrations and by rising concentrations of ADP and AMP. Citrate is a potent inhibitor of the enzyme, serving as a signal that the Krebs citric acid cycle is adequately supplied with fuel so that glycolysis can be slowed down or stopped. In addition to these sensitivities to metabolic intermediates and adenylates, PFK activity responds sharply to small changes in pH. Decreases in pH through the physiological pH range inhibit PFK, while increases in pH can strongly activate the enzyme [13–17]. It is apparent, then, that PFK and LDH (in its pyruvate reductase capacity) respond oppositely to changes in pH. Before discussing the implications of these opposing pH responses for the coordination of glycolytic activity, we must examine the mechanistic basis of the pH effects on PFK. We then will be in a strong position for understanding the overall bases of pH-induced changes in glycolytic flux rate and in the relative aerobic versus anaerobic poise of glycolysis. We will also see another clear case in which the advantages of alphastat regulation for the conservation of key protein characteristics can be observed in both short-term responses to rapid changes in T_B and in long-term evolutionary adaptation to temperature.

The influences of changes in pH and temperature on PFK activity are more complex than the effects discussed earlier for LDH. Nonetheless, the same basic principles given earlier concerning the benefits of alphastat regulation apply equally for both enzymes. The pH-induced changes in PFK activity (Fig. 6) are

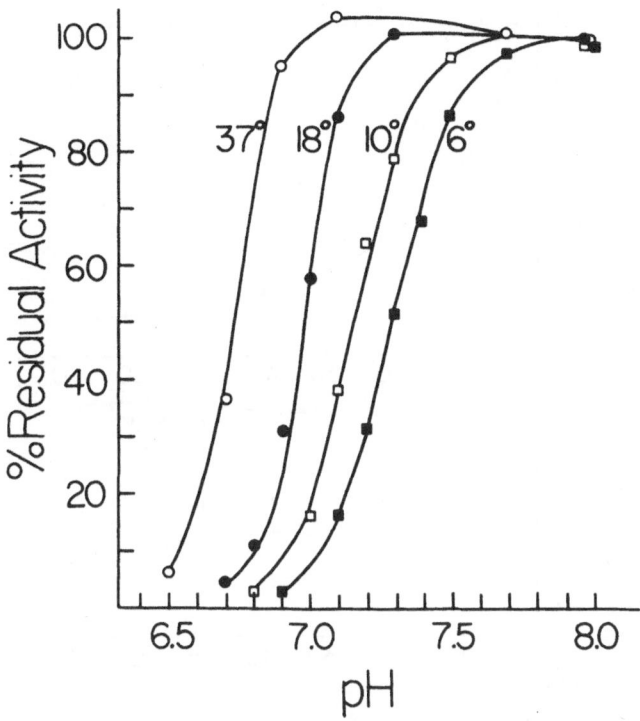

Fig. 6. The effects of 60-minute incubations at different pH and temperatures on the activity of phosphofructokinase purified from the squirrel, *Citellus beecheyi*. Aliquots of the enzyme were assayed at 25° C and pH 8.0. The figure is from Hand and Somero [17].

not a simple consequence of titration of active site histidine imidazole groups, as in the case for LDH, but instead derive from pH dependent changes in the subunit aggregation state of the enzyme (Fig. 7). PFK readily undergoes shifts between tetrameric and dimeric assembly states, and these alterations in subunit aggregation state are accompanied by 'on-off' changes in PFK activity [13–17]. Only the tetrameric form of the enzyme is catalytically active. The subunits of the dimer, while maintaining native conformation, have no enzymatic activity. Dimers that are generated by exposure of the enzyme to low pH can reassemble rapidly when the pH is raised, however, as shown in Fig. 7-C.

A strong interaction is noted between the effects of low temperature and low pH on PFK assembly state and activity (Figs. 6, 7). For example, at 6°C, the catalytic activity of the enzyme (Fig. 7-A) and the subunit aggregation state, as indicated by light scattering measurements (Fig. 7-B), are stable during prolonged incubation at pH 8.0. However, at an incubation pH of 7.1 at 6°C, loss of catalytic activity is rapid due to the dissociation of the active tetramers into inactive dimers; this dissociation is indicated by a fall in light scattering by the solution. These effects of changes in temperature and pH have been noted for PFKs from several vertebrate species [14–17], and the sharp responses of the

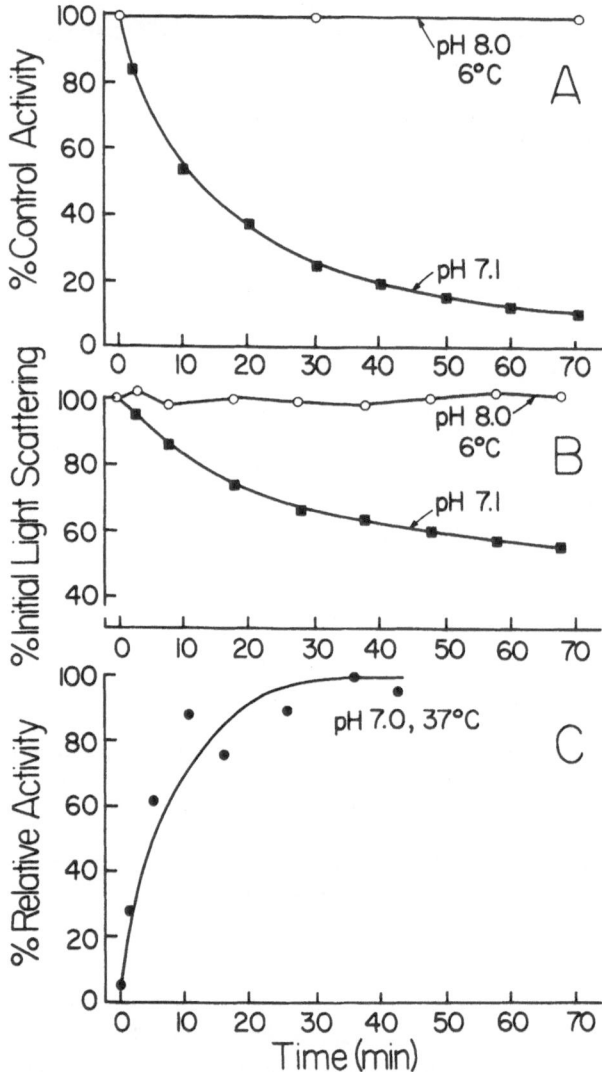

Fig. 7. A) Loss of PFK activity with time during incubation at pH 7.1 and 6° C. Activity is expressed as a percent of the activity of the enzyme incubated at pH 8.0 and 6°C. B) Change in light scattering during incubation of PFK at pH 7.1 and 6° C. Loss of light scattering reflects dissociation of the tetrameric form of the enzyme to the catalytically inactive dimer. C) Regain of activity of PFK that had been dissociated at low temperature and low pH. The regain of activity (= tetrameric state) is shown at pH 7.0 and 37° C. All data are for PFK of *C. beecheyi* [17].

enzyme from the squirrel, *Citellus beechevi*, illustrated in Figs. 6 and 7 appear to be general properties of vertebrate muscle PFKs.

Although the amino acid(s) in the PFK molecule that are responsible for the temperature and pH effects shown in Figs. 6 and 7 have not been determined, there is a strong basis for implicating one or more histidyl residues in these effects.

The residual activity curves shown in Fig. 6 bear a striking resemblance to histidyl imidazole titration curves. If at each temperature we equate the pH value at which fifty percent of the original activity is retained as an apparent pK for the residue being titrated, then the similarities between these 'titration' curves and actual imidazole titration curves are obvious. Thus, the apparent pK values so determined are close to the pK values for imidazole side-chains at the measurement temperatures (see Fig. 1), and the dependence of these apparent pK values on temperature (the apparent pK rises by 0.0186 pH units per degree Celsius fall in incubation temperature) is essentially the same as the temperature dependence of the pK of histidine imidazole groups (see Fig. 1). This is strong, albeit indirect, evidence that the temperature and pH effects on PFK derive from the titration of histidyl imidazole groups that are major effectors of the subunit aggregation state of the enzyme.

These very marked influences of pH and temperature on PFK have several important implications for our analysis of the enzymatic consequences of alphastat regulation. First, as in the case of LDH, the maintenance of pH_i near pK_{imid} renders PFK highly sensitive to small changes in pH_i, as might occur during transitions between rest and highly active locomotory states. The ability of pH_i values near the lower end of the physiological pH range for any given body temperature (see Fig. 1) to sharply reduce PFK activity (Fig. 6) and, thereby, the rate of glycolytic flux, may provide the cell with an important mechanism for preventing extreme acidification of the intracellular milieu under conditions of intense anaerobic function. That is, as excessive proton accumulation takes place during intense or prolonged bouts of anaerobic glycolysis, the inhibition of PFK will reduce, or fully curtail, glycolytic flux, and further acidifiction due to lactate production will be blocked.

A second implication of the pH and temperature effects on PFK assembly and activity is that glycolytic function at different body temperatures can be sustained only if an alphastat regulatory strategy is maintained. If T_B is decreased and pH_i is maintained constant, i.e., if pHstat conditions are maintained, the resulting acidotic state of the cytosol can lead to a strong depression in glycolytic activity due to the combined influences of rate deceleration per se due to falling temperature and disassembly with loss of activity of PFK.

In this context it is interesting to consider an extreme case of low-body-temperature acidosis that occurs under natural conditions. In small mammalian hibernators, e.g., squirrels, several tissues, including skeletal muscle, retain a pH_i close to the value found under normothermic conditions (near 37° C) even when T_B falls to 2–4° C [18; see Chapter 2 by Malan]. Under these conditions of low temperature acidosis, our in vitro data (Figs. 6 and 7) suggest that PFK activity will be completely abolished, i.e., muscle glycolysis will be fully inhibited in the hibernating state. In fact, for at least one species of hibernator, *Citellus lateralis*, where the appropriate measurements of muscle glycogen content have been made, there was a complete conservation of muscle glycogen stores throughout

the hibernation period [19]. Retention of muscle glycogen stores during hibernation seems adaptive, of course, since the restoration of normothermic temperature by shivering, and the initiation of locomotory activity following arousal will
both depend on a capacity for active muscle glycogenolysis [17]. In many small
mammalian hibernators, then, a 'failure' to maintain alphastat pH regulation in
muscle during hibernation may yield important benefits.

It is interesting that heart and liver differ in their pH regulatory strategy during
hibernation from what is found in skeletal muscle. While the pH_i of cardiac
muscle of non-hibernating mammals reflects the trends of extracellular fluid
alterations in pH [20], the hibernator heart, and liver as well, follow an alphastat
pattern in the face of pHstat regulation of the extracellular fluid [18, 21]. This
observation suggests that hibernators possess specialized regulatory mechanisms
for the extrusion of protons from these tissues which preserve net protein charge
state as in typical ectothermic species. The efforts made by small mammalian
hibernators to maintain alphastat conditions in organs that continue to serve
critical functions during deep hibernation would seem to have an important
message for physicians seeking to establish optimal physiological conditions
during hypothermic surgical procedures.

PFK-temperature-pH interactions: An evolutionary perspective

We saw in the case of pH and temperature effects on LDH that the significance of
alphastat regulation applies in both short-term and evolutionary time courses.
We proposed that the conservation of critical enzymatic properties, like K_m
values and structural integrity, in the face of varying body temperatures would be
facilitated by the alphastat regulatory scheme in the cases of rapid changes in the
body temperature of an individual organism and on broader, interspecific scales.
For PFK, the importance of alphastat regulation on an evolutionary time frame is
clearly apparent. As shown by the data of Fig. 6, subjecting PFK from mammalian muscle to the low body temperatures characteristic of many ectothermic
species leads to a complete, or near-complete, loss of activity under pHstat
conditions. If pHstat regulation were to pertain in nature, then it is apparent that
amino acid replacements in the PFK molecule would be necessary to ensure
continued PFK function in low-body-temperature species. Alphastat regulation
would seem to preclude the need for such amino acid substitutions in the case of
PFK structural integrity. Therefore, we believe it is appropriate to argue that
alphastat regulation, in a sense, 'simplifies' biochemical evolution, by minimizing
or eliminating the requirement for amino acid substitutions that would be required, under pHstat regimens, to offset the perturbing effects of low temperature and low pH. In this context it is pertinent to stress that many studies of the
phenomenon of 'cold lability' of proteins suffer from the shortcoming that the
experiments did not take into account the possible interactions of low tempera-

ture and low pH [7, 22]. The putative 'cold lability' of many proteins reported in the literature may, in reality, be but a manifestation of the pH sensitivities of protein structure. The denaturing influences of reductions in experimental temperature may, in many of these instances, be carried out through increases in the protonation states of histidyl imidazole groups, as has been proposed for PFK.

pH optima of enzymatic reactions versus temperature

In view of the effects of changes in pH and temperature on the K_m values and structural integrities of enzymes discussed above, it is appropriate to inquire how the pH optima of enzymatic reactions, i.e., the dependence of reaction velocity on pH, vary with measurement temperature. This topic has been treated in an elegant fashion by Wilson [23, 24], who has discussed not only temperature effects on enzymes arising from imidazole groups, but also from other ionizable groups, e.g., sulphydryl groups. Despite the interest in this subject, however, there are extremely few data available which show how the optimal pH of an enzymatic reaction varies with temperature. Furthermore, many of the existing data are difficult to interpret because the effects of temperature and pH on V_{max} and K_m have not been distinguished. Nonetheless, it is worth examining the available information in an attempt to expand our understanding of the role of alphastat regulation in maintaining enzymatic function at different temperatures.

Hazel and colleagues [25] have gathered the largest data set dealing with this question. They examined both cytosolic and mitochondrial enzymes in their study, and the trends they noted are shown in Fig. 8, which also includes data calculated from other published experiments [26, 27]. All of the enzymes so examined showed a rise in pH optimum with decreasing temperature, the slope of this relationship varying somewhat among different classes of enzymes (the footnote to Fig. 8 lists these slopes). For some of the enzymes, the change in optimal pH with temperature was very close to the expected effect of a temperature-dependent shift in the pK of an imidazole side-chain. It is noteworthy, too, that the pH optima of the mitochondrial enzymes were higher, at any given measurement temperature, than those of the cytosolic enzymes. This observation is, of course, consistent with the occurrence of a higher pH in the mitochondrial matrix than in the cytosol. Although it is not clear if histidyl imidazole groups are responsible for the temperature and pH effects noted for these different enzymes, it should not be concluded that the higher pH optima for the mitochondrial enzymes reflect the role of a side-chain other than the imidazole group. The pK values of imidazole groups are subject to wide variation, depending on the local microenvironment in which they are located [9], so the pH responses of both the cytosolic and the mitochondrial matrix enzymes could be reflections of imidazole effects.

Two additional studies show that pH optima can be the result of complex

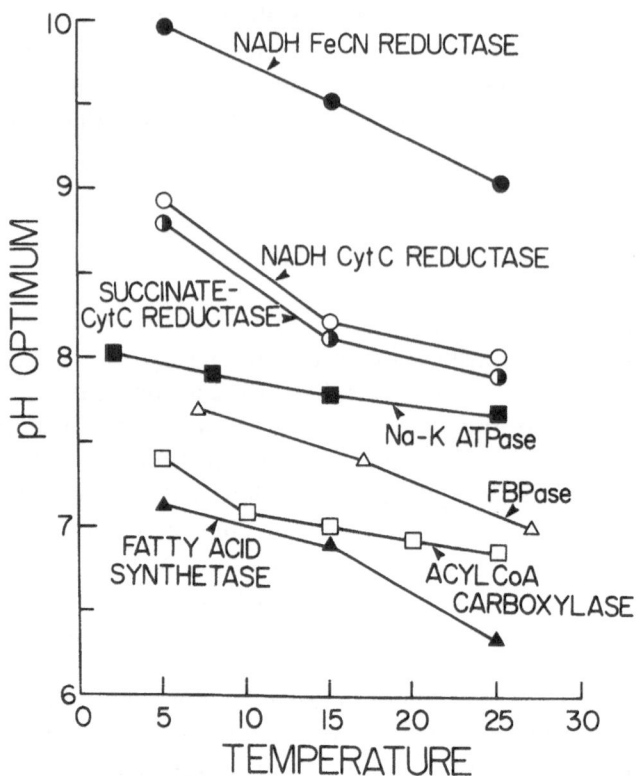

Fig. 8. Influence of measurement temperature on the pH optimum of several enzymatic reactions. The number in parentheses after the name of the enzyme listed below is the average slope of the pH optimum *versus* temperature relationship. Data for the mitochondrial enzymes, NADH ferricyanide reductase (−0.040), NADH cytochrome c reductase (−0.044), and succinate cytochrome c reductase (−0.044) are from [25]. Data for Na-K-ATPase (−0.017) are from [26]. Data on fructose-1,6-bisphosphatase (FBPase) (−0.033) are from [27]. Data for acylCoA carboxylase (−0.027) and fatty acid synthetase (−0.0282) are from [25].

effects that clearly involve more than the titration of a single imidazole group (Fig. 9). The studies of Park and Hong [26] on toad skin Na-K-ATPase and of Rosenmann *et al.* [27] on carp muscle fructose-1,6-bisphosphatase (FBPase) showed that extremely sharp pH optima having pronounced temperature dependence characterize these two enzymes. For both enzymes, decreases in temperature led to higher pH optima, but the slopes of these relationships were quite different. For the Na-K-ATPase of toad skin, the slope (pH optima versus measurement temperature) was approximately −0.017, while for FBPase the slope was approximately −0.033. In both studies care was taken to measure true V_{max} values at the different temperature and pH values, so these data probably reflect pH and temperature influences on the conversion of substrate to product, rather than on the initial binding of substrates.

Despite the apparent contribution of titratable groups besides imidazole to

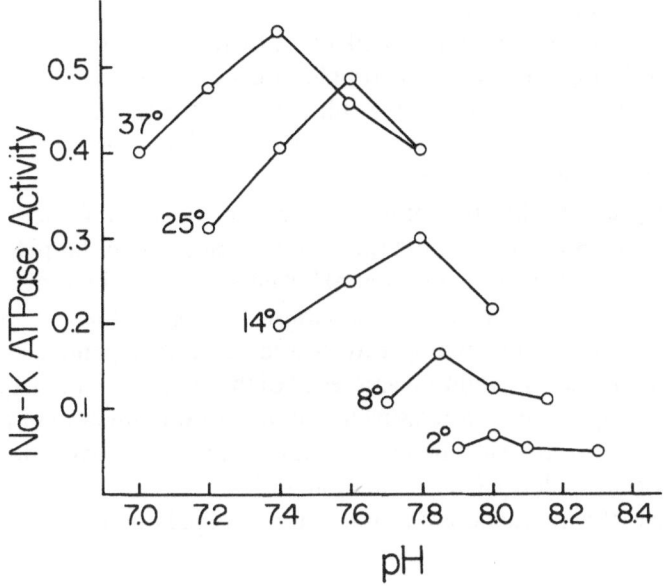

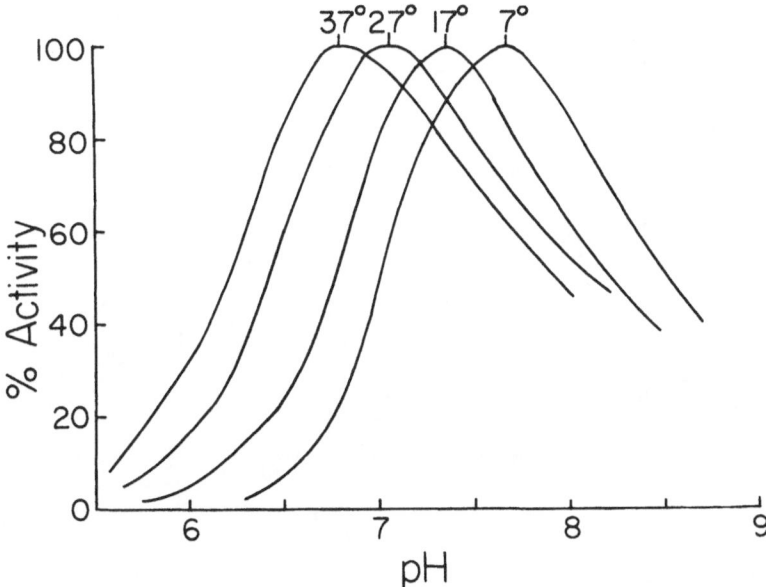

Fig. 9. Upper frame. Effect of temperature on the pH optimum of the Na-K-ATPase reaction of toad skin. Data are from [26]. Lower frame. Effect of temperature on the pH optimum of the fructose 1,6-bisphosphatase (FBPase) reaction of carp muscle. Data are from [27].

these pH/temperature effects on Na-K-ATPase and FBPase, as suggested by the bell-shaped titration curves and, for FBPase, by the slope of the relationship of optimal pH to temperature, the favorable effect of alphastat regulation on the conservation of enzymatic activity is still apparent for these two enzymes. For both enzymes, the rise in pH_i with decreasing body temperature leads to a stabilization of enzymatic activity in the face of temperature change. In Fig. 10 we illustrate, diagramatically, the differences in temperature effects on enzymatic reaction rate which result from the functioning, under alphastat pH_i conditions, of two enzymes for which the optimal pH is either independent of temperature (left frame of figure) or varies with temperature in approximate agreement with pK of imidazole. Note how significantly the temperature dependence (Q_{10}) of the latter enzyme's reaction is reduced as a result of the enzyme's shift in pH optimum with varying temperature. Note as well that alphastat regulation of pH_i leads to higher Q_{10} values for the enzyme having a temperature-independent optimal pH than would occur under pHstat regulation.

In summary, the interactions of temperature and pH on the rates of enzymatic

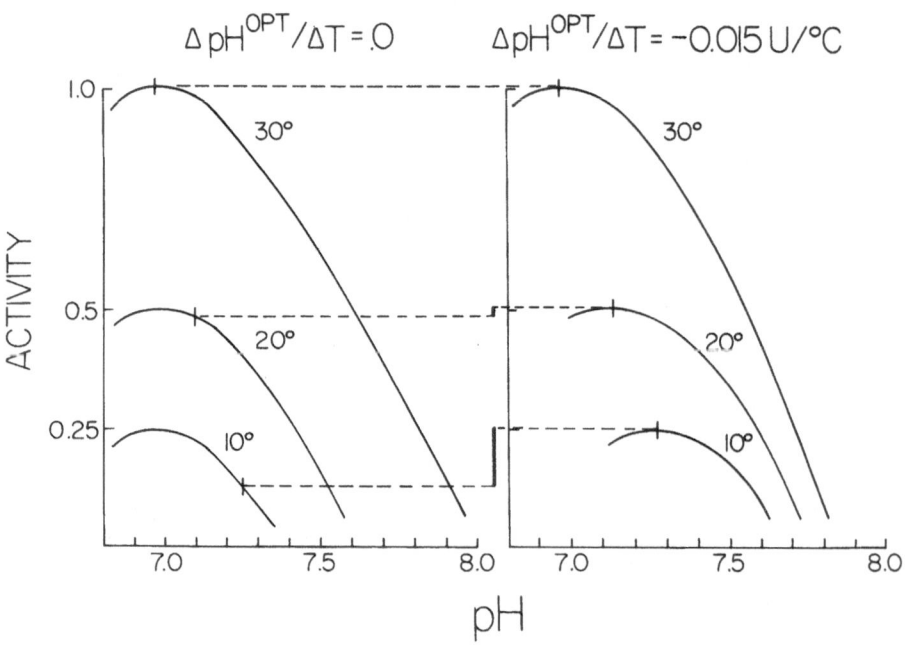

Fig. 10. Effect of temperature on the activities of enzymes having either a temperature-insensitive pH optimum (pH^{opt}) (left panel), or a pH optimum that decreases by −0.015 pH units per degree Celsius rise in temperature (right panel). For both enzymes, a change in cytosol pH of −0.015 pH unit per degree Celsius increase in temperature is assumed. Note that the rightward displacement of the activity versus pH curves for the enzyme having the temperature-dependent pH optimum leads to a reduction in the effect of temperature on reaction velocity. The difference in reaction rate between the two enzymes is shown (at 20° C and 10° C) by the dark vertical line connected by dashed lines between the two panels. Figure is from [9].

activity, as well as on the integrity of enzyme structure, argue convincingly that alphastat regulation is of crucial importance in conserving the structural and functional properties of enzymes and other proteins in the face of varying body temperature. Our task now is to see how more complex metabolic systems, e.g., the metabolism of intact organs, benefit from the alphastat strategy of pH regulation.

pH effects on glycolysis: Comparisons of in vitro and in vivo studies

It is a relatively simple task to study enzymes in vitro and use the resulting data to make predictions about metabolic effects in vivo. Demonstrating the validity of these predictions frequently is difficult, however, and many biochemical hypotheses may have a long lifetime in the theoretical realm before they are subject to rigorous in vivo examination. Fortunately, excellent data are available for testing certain of the predictions made in the preceding sections of this article. In particular we can draw on studies in which experimentally induced changes in intramuscular pH have been correlated with changes both in total glycolytic flux (as we predict from pH effects on PFK) and in the relative channeling of carbon between pyruvate and lactate (effects we predict based on the pH reponses of LDH). Williamson and colleagues [28] have studied the effects of induced acidosis on the metabolism of mammalian cardiac muscle at 37° C. A key finding of their studies was that changes in pH_i altered both the total activity of the glycolytic pathway and the relative partitioning of carbon flow between pyruvate and lactate. When pH_i was decreased from 6.95 to 6.57 by reducing the pH of the perfusion medium from 7.4 to 6.6, the total flux through the glycolytic sequence decreased by 71 percent. Simultaneously, the percentage of carbon accumulating as lactate rose from 31 to 76, and the lactate: pyruvate ratio increased 10-fold. These are precisely the effects we would predict from the in vitro responses of PFK and LDH to pH changes over this pH range.

In addition to these changes in glycolytic rate and lactate/pyruvate balance, Williamson et al. [28] noted physiological changes that displayed pH responses similar to those found in studies of PFK under in vitro conditions. For instance, the shift in left ventricular pressure development with changes in pH_i followed a pattern almost indentical to that noted for PFK activity as a function of pH, as shown in Fig. 6 (37° C curve) (cf. Fig. 3 of Williamson et al. [28]).

Other studies of pH influences on cardiac function have examined the interactions of pH and T_B on heart performance. In their study of canine hearts maintained either under classical acid-base management strategy of constant pH of 7.4, or under alphastat conditions, Swain et al. [29] showed that the decrease in electrical fibrillation threshold noted under the former experimental condition did not occur under alphastat conditions. An improvement in heart performance under alphastat conditions during hypothermia was also shown by McConnell et *al.* [30]. Using pH conditions that were even slightly more alkaline than true alphastat conditions, these workers showed an improvement, relative to pHstat conditions, in the heart's capacity to utilize lactate, in coronary blood flow, and in the ability of the left ventricle to generate force when challenged by balloon inflation in the aorta.

The results of physiological studies are, in general, in good agreement with the results of, and predictions based on, studies of enzymes in vitro. This conclusion is emphasized by Wiliamson *et al.* [28] who point out that, in addition to LDH and PFK, whose pH responses are well studied and which provide at least a partial mechanistic basis for explaining the organ-level effects they noted in their study of heart function, several other enzymes of energy metabolism also display pH responses that are in agreement with the results of the organ-level study. For example, decreases in pH inhibit citrate synthase, which catalyzes the entry of Acetyl-CoA into the Krebs citric acid cycle, and pyruvate dehydrogenase, the enzyme complex which is responsible for generating Acetyl-CoA. Thus, aerobic metabolism, like anaerobic glycolysis, can be sharply affected by small (0.1 to 0.3 unit) changes in pH_i, as, indeed, the data of Hazel *et al.* [25; Fig. 8] also suggest. It is noteworthy in this context that, in a study of oxygen consumption by isolated, perfused canine hind limb, Harken [31] observed that oxygen consumption rate was linearly related to the pH of the perfusion medium; over the range of 6.95 to 7.65, oxygen comsumption increased regularly with rising pH.

Alphastat regulation and the maintenance of pH gradients.

Up to this point in our discussion we have focused largely on the benefits of alphastat regulation for protein systems in which histidyl imidazole groups play major roles in establishing structure and/or function. An additional benefit of alphastat regulation has recently been proposed by Yacoe [32], who has presented indirect evidence that stabilization of the pH gradient across the inner membrane of the mitochondrion is favored by alphastat regulation, and stabilization of this pH gradient fosters a reduction in the temperature sensitivity of succinate oxidation by mitochondria.

Yacoe [32] studied the influences of temperature, pH, and P_{CO_2} on the oxidation of succinate by mitochondria isolated from liver of the desert iguana, *Dipsosaurus dorsalis.* The effect of succinate concentration on oxygen consumption by the mitochondria closely obeyed Michaelis-Menten kinetics, so the effects of temperature, pH, and P_{CO_2} on both the K_m and V_{max} of succinate oxidation could be dertermined. As expected, temperature affected the V_{max} of the reaction, and the Q_{10} observed was slightly greater than two. Neither the pH nor the P_{CO_2} of the medium influenced V_{max}, however. In contrast, the K_m of succinate was influenced, in a complex fashion, by all three variables. The pertinent findings for our discussion are that large differences in the temperature dependence of K_m were found between alphastat and pHstat regulatory strategies, and that these different responses of the K_m of succinate to temperature led to significantly different Q_{10} values for succinate oxidation under physiologically realistic conditions of succinate concentration.

Figure 11 presents these findings in a simplified manner, showing how the Q_{10} of succinate oxidation varies, as a function of succinate concentration, under alphastat and pHstat conditions. The reason for expressing the temperature effects as a function of succinate concentration is that, in the mitochondrion, succinate concentration are apt to be well below saturation for the reaction [cf. 32]. Thus, as discussed earlier in the case of the LDH reaction, effects on the K_m of the reaction can lead to large changes in reaction velocity, even though the V_{max} of the reaction is not affected by the experimental variable, pH in this case. Under alphastat pH regulation, the Q_{10} of succinate oxidation at physiological succinate concentrations lies somewhere between approximately 2.2 and 2.4, whereas under pHstat conditions, the Q_{10} may rise to values greater than 3 (Fig. 11).

In discussing these interesting findings, Yacoe [32] stresses that the proposed advantages of alphastat regulation to this system are not likely to be the result of simple effects on histidyl imidazole charge. Rather, the complex effects of changes in pH and P_{CO_2} argue strongly for a role of alphastat regulation in

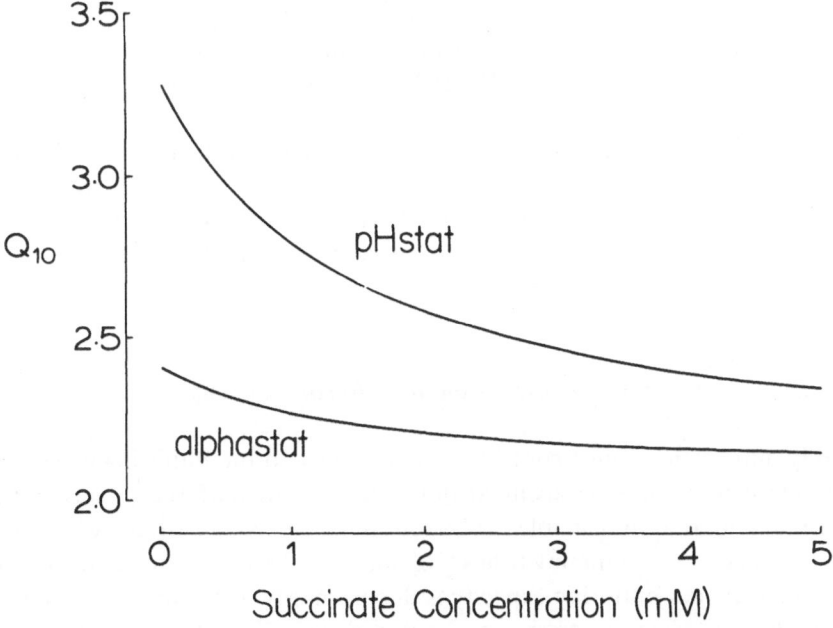

Fig. 11. Q_{10} of succinate oxidation by mitochondria isolated from liver of *Dipsosaurus dorsalis* shown as a function of succinate concentration, under alphastat and pHstat regimens. The Q_{10}s are for the temperature range of 25 to 40° C. The different responses of Q_{10} to succinate concentration under the two pH regimens are a reflection of temperature and pH influences on the K_m of succinate (see text for discussion). The figure is modified after [32].

stabilizing the pH gradient that exists across the inner mitochondrial membrane. For example, the opposite effects of a decrease in pH and an increase in P_{CO_2} on the K_m of succinate observed by Yacoe [32] show that more than a histidyl imidazole protonation event is involved when either of these acid-base variables changes the K_m of succinate. All of the observed effects of pH and P_{CO_2} were consistent, however, with effects on the transmembrane pH gradient. Decreases in medium pH would be expected to increase this gradient, while increases in medium P_{CO_2} would decrease the gradient, since CO_2 behaves as a permeable weak acid that can cross the inner mitochondrial membrane, and lead to acidification of the mitochondrial matrix. Earlier studies using rat liver mitochondria [33, 34] showed that changes in the pH gradient across the inner mitochondrial membrane led to significant changes in the K_m of succinate. Thus, any condition, such as alphastat regulation, which can stabilize this gradient will stabilize the K_m of succinate. And, in the case of succinate oxidation by mitochondria of ectothermic species like *D. dorsalis*, stabilization of K_m was shown to greatly reduce the Q_{10} of the reaction (Fig. 11).

The lower Q_{10} values found for succinate oxidation by mitochondria under alphastat conditions, compared to pHstat conditions (Fig. 11), resemble the findings obtained by McConnell *et al.* [30] in their studies of oxygen consumption by canine hearts under these two pH regimens. The Q_{10} values found in this study under alphastat and pHstat regimens were approximately 2 and 4, respectively.

In summary, although the mechanisms by which alphastat pH regulation might achieve a stabilization of the pH gradient across the inner membrane of the mitochondrion are not known, from the evidence provided by Yacoe [32] it appears that the conservation of this critical property of the mitochondrion may be another significant effect of alphastat regulation. And, as Yacoe stresses, these findings show that the physiological benefits that accrue from alphastat regulation may be manifested in systems where more complex pH effects are involved than relatively simple titration effects on histidyl imidazole groups.

Alphastat regulation and conservation of buffering capacity

Histidyl imidazole groups contribute significantly to the buffering capacities of both intracellular and extracellular fluids. In strongly buffered tissues, e.g., the breast muscles of birds capable of vigorous bursts of flying [35], the white epaxial muscles of actively swimming fishes [36], and muscles of certain diving mammals [36], the elevated buffering capacity is due primarily to the histidine-containing dipeptides, anserine, carnosine, and ophidine [35, 37, 38], or, in rare cases, to high concentrations of free histidine [38].

The prevalent role of imidazole buffers in biological fluids has some interesting ramifications for the discussion of pH regulatory strategies. Indeed, where imidazole buffers are present at extremely high concentrations, the physico-chemical buffering provided by imidazole groups may be the principal determinant of the response of the pH of a fluid compartment to a change in temperature. In fluid compartments where imidazole buffering is by far the dominant component of the buffer system, then, there will be no change in the tissue's buffering capacity as body temperature varies.

In other tissues, where buffering by other components, e.g., phosphate compounds, also makes a significant contribution to total buffering capacity, shifts in T_B will not lead directly to alphastat pH patterns. To achieve an alphastat pH value, physiological regulation may be required [cf. Chapter 2, this volume]. Alphastat pH regulation will not only conserve the key protein features discussed throughout this essay, but also will preserve the buffering capacity of the imidazole fraction of the buffer system. Suffice it to say that the benefits of alphastat regulation are likely to extend to all systems in which imidazole groups play important roles.

Intracellular pH increases and metabolic activation

To conclude our discussion of the consequences of alphastat regulation for protein function, we shall consider diverse situations in which the restoration of an alphastat pH value in an acidotic system leads to a substantial metabolic activation. These instances of metabolic activation, which have been observed in a varied suite of prokaryotic and eukaryotic systems, offer an especially strong basis for concluding that alphastat regulation is of importance among different physiological systems, and among phylogenetically diverse organisms.

Due in significant measure to the development of accurate, non-invasive techniques for measuring intracellular pH, notably nuclear magnetic resonance (NMR) methods, there has been a proliferation of studies of pH_i in recent years. Many of the most important of these studies are discussed in the recent symposium volume edited by Nuccitelli and Deamer [40]. One of the most interesting discoveries that has been made in these investigations of intracellular pH values is that, in a diverse array of metabolic systems, transition from an acidotic condition to an alphastat pH value is marked by a large increase in metabolic activity. While this response to an increase in pH has customarily, and misleadingly, been referred to as metabolic activation due to 'alkalinization,' we emphasize that the final pH of the activated system is not alkaline, but rather is near the pH predicted by alphastat theory. That is, during the activation of metabolism there is an increase in pH_i, but this increase must be viewed as an elimination of an acidotic state, not the establishment of an alkalotic state. Unfortunately, most workers dealing with these phenomena have not discussed their findings in terms of alphastat theory.

Among the systems in which the elimination of an acidotic state has been correlated with a sharp rise in the function of the system are: respiration in

78

developing echinoderm embryos, protein synthesis rates in embryos, metabolic function in brine shrimp embryos after cyst hydration, activation of bacterial metabolism following spore germination, and, as already discussed, muscle glycolysis. The review of Nuccitelli and Heiple [40] provides an up-to-date list of these phenomena. The finding that so many different types of metabolic processes are activated by the elimination of an acidotic state, and the establishment of an alphastat pH value, argues for the widespread occurrence of pH-mediated control of metabolic processes, and for the importance of alphastat pH regulation in conserving metabolic capacities. Furthermore, the finding that these activation phenomena usually involve pH increases of only 0.1 to 0.4 pH unit shows that pH decreases of only a few tenths of a pH unit from the alphastat state are adequate to promote large alterations in metabolic function. As we emphasized in the section on mitochondrial function and pH gradients, the stabilizing benefits of alphastat regulation on metabolic function may be due to a variety of effects, ranging from direct influences on the protonation state of histidyl imidazole groups to more complex effects, such as those proposed to involve the conservation of pH gradients across membranes.

These pervasive effects of small changes in pH_i on so many different metabolic processes, in widely different organisms, would seem to supply a compelling raison d'etre for alphastat regulation. The discovery that severe depression of metabolism can accompany entry into the acidotic state should serve as a clear warning to clinicians who, during clinical procedures using hypothermia, must decide which pH regulatory strategy to follow. The study of comparative physiology has shown us that the internal milieu of the organism represents the product of an elaborate evolutionary history [7, 41]. Only when the properties of the internal milieu are conserved within quite narrow limits is the well being of the organism maintained. The lessons of comparative physiology and enlightened medical practice thus argue that an alphastat regulatory strategy is of ubiquitous importance, whether the organism is in its natural habitat, or in a clinical setting.

Acknowledgements

The development of many of the ideas discussed in this article reflects the stimulation and insights provided by discussions with Drs. Hermann Rahn and R. Blake Reeves. Certain of the studies reviewed in this article were supported by National Science Foundation grants PCM80-01949 and PCM83-00983 to G.N. Somero and PCM82-04545 to F.N. White.

References

1. Reeves RB, Rahn H: Patterns in vertebrate acid-base regulation. In: *Evolution of Respiratory Processes: A Comparative Approach*, Wood SC, Lenfant C (eds). Marcel Dekker, New York, 1979: 225–252.
2. Reeves RB: The interaction of body temperature and acid-base balance in ectothermic vertebrates. Ann Rev Physiol 39: 559–586, 1977.
3. Rahn H, Reeves RB, Howell BJ: Hydrogen ion regulation, temperature and evolution. Am Rev Respir Dis 112: 165–172, 1975.
4. Rahn H, Howell BJ: The OH^-/H^+ concept of acid-base balance: historical development. Respir Physiol 33: 91–97, 1978
5. Reeves RB: An imidazole alphastat hypothesis for vertebrate acid-base regulation: tissue carbon dioxide content and body temperature in bullfrogs. Respir Physiol 14: 219–236, 1972.
6. Fersht A: Enzyme Structure and Mechanism. W.H. Freeman, San Francisco, 1977.
7. Hochachka PW, Somero GN: Biochemical Adaptation. Princeton University Press, Princeton, 1984.
8. Yancey PH, Somero GN: Temperature dependence of intracellular pH: its role in the conservation of pyruvate apparent K_m values of vertebrate lactate dehydrogenases. J Comp Physiol 125: 129–134, 1978.
9. Somero GN: pH-temperature interactions on proteins: principles of optimal pH and buffer system design. Mar Biol Lett 2: 163–178, 1980.
10. Somero GN: Enviromental adaptation of proteins. Comp Biochem Physiol 76A: 621–633, 1984.
11. Walsh PJ, Somero GN: Interactions among pyruvate concentration, pH, and K_m of pyruvate in determining *in vivo* Q_{10} values of the lactate dehydrogenase reaction. Can J Zool 60: 1293–1299, 1982.
12. Blayo MC, Lecompte Y, Pocidalo JJ: Control of acid-base status during hypothermia in man. Respir Physiol 42: 287–298, 1980.
13. Uyeda K: Phosphofructokinase. Adv Enzymol Relat Areas Mol Biol 48: 193–244, 1979.
14. Bock PE, Frieden C: Phosphofructokinase.I. Mechanism of the pH-dependent inactivation and reactivation of the rabbit muscle enzyme. J Biol Chem 251: 5630–5636, 1976.
15. Bock PE, Frieden C: Phosphofructokinase. II. Role of ligands in pH-dependent structural changes of the rabbit muscle enzyme. J Biol Chem 251: 5637–5643, 1976.
16. Hand SC, Somero GN: Urea and methylamine effects on rabbit muscle phosphofructokinase. Catalytic stability and aggregation state as a function of pH and temperature. J Biol Chem 257: 734–741, 1982.
17. Hand SC, Somero GN: Phosphofructokinase of the hibernator, *Citellus beecheyi*: temperature and pH regulation of activity *via* influences on the tetramer-dimer equilibrium. Physiol Zool 56: 380–388, 1983.
18. Malan A: Enzyme regulation, metabolic rate, and acid-base status in hiberation. In: Animals and Environmental Fitness: Physiological and Biochemical Aspects of Adaptations and Ecology. Proceedings of the First Conference of the European Society for Comparative Physiology and Biochemistry. Vol. 1, Gilles J (ed). Pergamon, New York, 1980: 187–501.
19. Zimmerman ML: Carbohydrate status, plasma glucose, and torpor duration in hibernating golden-mantled ground squirrels: effects of carbohydrate loading with odd-numbered fatty acids. J Comp Physiol 147: 129–135, 1982.
20. Jacobus WE, Pores IH, Lucas SK, Kallman CH, Weisfeldt ML, Flaherty JT: The role of intracellular pH in the control of normal and ischemic myocardial contractility: A ^{31}P nuclear magnetic resonance and mass spectrometry study. In: Intracellular pH: Its Measurement, Regulation, and Utilization in Cellular Function, Nuccitelli R, Deamer DW (eds). Allen R. Liss, New York, 1982: 537–565.
21. Malan A: Respiration and acid-base state in hiberation. In: Hibernation and Torpor in Mammals

and Birds, Lyman CP, Willis JS, Malan A, Wang LCH (eds). Academic Press, New York, 1983: 237–282.

22. Beyer RF: Effects of low temperature on cold-sensitive enzymes from mammalian tissues. In: Hibernation-Hypothermia: Perspectives and Challenges, South FE, Hannon JP, Willis JR, Pengelley ET, Alpert NR (eds). Elsevier, Amsterdam, 1972: 17–54.

23. Wilson TL: Interrelations between pH and temperature for the catalytic rate of the M_4 isozyme of lactate dehydrogenase (EC 1.1.1.27) from goldfish (*Carassius auratus* L). Arch Biochem Biophys 179: 378–390, 1977.

24. Wilson TL: Theoretical analysis of the effects of two pH regulation patterns on the temperature sensitivities of biological systems in nonhomeothermic animals. Arch Biochem Biophys 182: 409–419, 1977.

25. Hazel JR, Garlick WS, Sellner PA: The effects of assay temperature upon the pH optima of enzymes from poikilotherms: A test of the imidazole alphastat hypothesis. J Comp Physiol 123: 97–104, 1978.

26. Park YS, Hong SK: Properties of toad skin Na-K-ATPase with special reference to effect of temperature. Am J Physiol 231: 1356–1363, 1976.

27. Rosenmann E, Gonzalez AM, Hein S, Marcus F: Carp (*Cyprinus carpio*) muscle fructose 1,6-bisphosphatase: purification and some properties. Comp Biochem Physiol 58B: 291–295, 1977.

28. Williamson JR, Safer B, Rich T, Schaffer S, Kobayashi K: Effects of acidosis on myocardial contractility and metabolism. Acta Med Scan Suppl 587: 95–111, 1975.

29. Swain JA, White FN, Peters RM: The effect of pH on the hypothermic fibrillation threshold. J Thorac Cardio Surg 87: 445–451, 1984.

30. McConnell DH, White FN, Nelson RL, Goldstein SM, Maloney JV, DeLand EC, Buckberg GD: Importance of 'alkalosis' in maintenance of ideal blood pH during hypothermia. Surg Forum 26: 263–265, 1975.

31. Harken AH: Hydrogen ion concentration and oxygen uptake in an isolated canine hindlimb. J Appl Physiol 40: 1–5, 1976.

32. Yacoe ME: Temperature and acid-base effects on the metabolism of isolated hepatic mitochondria of the desert iguana, *Dipsosaurus dorsalis* . Submitted for publication.

33. Quagliariello E, Palmieri F: Control of succinate oxidation by succinate uptake by rat liver mitochondria. Eur J Biochem 4: 20–27, 1968.

34. Quagliariello E, Palmieri F, Prezioso G, Klingenberg M: Kinetics of succinate uptake by rat liver mitochondria. FEBS Lett. 4: 251–254, 1969.

35. Burton RF: Intracellular buffering. Respir Physiol 33: 51–58, 1978.

36. Castellini MA, Somero GN: Buffering capacity of vertebrate muscle: Correlations with potentials for anaerobic function. J Comp Physiol 143: 191–198, 1981.

37. Crush KG: Carnosine and related substances in animal tissues. Comp Biochem Physiol 34: 3–30, 1970.

38. Abe H: Distribution of free L-histidine and related dipeptides in the muscle of freshwater fishes. Comp Biochem Physiol 76B: 35–39, 1983.

39. Nuccitelli R, Deamer DW (eds): Intracellular pH: Its Measurement, Regulation, and Utilization in Cellular Functions. Allen R. Liss, New York, 1982.

40. Nuccitelli R, Heiple JM: Summary of the evidence and discussion concerning the involvement of pH_i in the control of cellular functions. In: Intracellular pH: Its Measurement, Regulation, and Utilization in Cellular Function, Nuccitelli R, Deamer DW (eds). New York, Allen R. Liss, New York, 1982: 567–586.

41. White FN, Somero GN: Acid-base regulation and phospholipid adaptations to temperature: Time courses and physiological significance of modifying the milieu for protein function. Physiol Rev 62: 40–90, 1982.

Clinical applications

5. Acid-base management during hypothermic circulatory arrest for cardiac surgery

HENRY SWAN

Abstract

Four fundamental strategies for acid-base management during hypothermic cardio-pulmonary by-pass (H-CPBP) are pH-stat, P_{CO_2}-stat, alpha-stat, and respiratory alkalosis. For H-CPBP in man, the blood is diluted with saline solution to HCT 20% (β is about 20 slykes). On the logC-T graph pH and P_{CO_2} lines are both horizontal. This graph closely approximates the human situation.

The heart and brain, both undergoing prolonged ischemia, are the special determinants of acid-base strategy during H-CPBP. Extensive analysis of available literature documents these opinions:

(1) Since acidosis is myotixic per se, excess CO_2 is deleterious to heart function. Prevention of ischemic acidosis by deliberate alkalosis before circulatory arrest, treatment by buffered alkaline cardiopreservative perfusion, and instant restoration with pH 7.8 reperfusion, are the keys to preservation and restoration of myocardial function.

(2) Although CO_2 does dilate cerebral vessels, there is no evidence that this practice increases cerebral tolerance to ischemia. Periods of total circulatory arrest in excess of 40 minutes should be avoided.

Since alpha-stat plots are invariant with buffer strengths, and the strategy has constant meter readings regardless of temperature, the use of temperature corrected blood gas samples for monitoring acid-base status is undesirable. Hyperventilation alkalosis can also be easily achieved with such data by use of the LogC-T nomogram. This management strategy is strongly recommended.

In an attempt to clarify possible options in the clinical management of hypothermia, Kindig et al. [1] have shown by graphic analysis the effect of various strategies on pH and P_{CO_2} between 37° and 17° C when T_{CO_2} (total carbon dioxide content) is held constant or is varied by the addition of CO_2 to the system or its removal by ventilation. Their model was a binary buffer system originally described by Rahn and Reeves [2] containing 130 mM/l of imidazole and 24.5 mM/l of CO_2. This system has a buffer strength of 44 slykes (mM/Δ1pH).[1] In this graph,

1. Buffer strength usually means the non-bicarbonate buffering capacity expressed as titration of a specific amount of acid or alkali per change of 1 unit of pH (mM/Δ1pH).

the pH isopleths were shown as slanting dotted lines and $\Delta pH/^\circ C$ was only .012.

This graphic analysis allowed a clearcut demonstration of four strategies for acid-base management of a patient undergoing hypothermic cardio-pulmonary bypass (H-CPBP) surgery. These four strategies were:

1) constant in vivo pH (pH-stat); this strategy is achieved by hypoventilation with 3–7% CO_2 added to the respiratory gas mixture.

2) constant in vivo P_{CO_2}; slightly less CO_2 is added to the respiratoy gases. Both of these strategies result in severe respiratory acidosis.

3) constant in vivo T_{CO_2} (alpha-stat); this strategy throughout the entire temperature range graphed, 37 to 17° C, results in constant 37° meter readings of pH 7.4 and of P_{CO_2} 40 torr. It has been described as alpha-stat [3, 75]; and represents biological neutrality at any temperature. At 17°, the in vivo pH is 7.72 and P_{CO_2} is 14.4; the meter reads 7.4, and 40 torr respectively. This is the strategy which keeps OH^-/H^+, alpha imidazole and protein charge state constant.

4) decreased in vivo T_{CO_2}; by vigorous hyperventilation the in vivo pH at 17° may be forced to approximate 7.9 with P_{CO_2} at about 6 torr. The meter will read pH 7.61 and P_{CO_2} 17. This is severe respiratory alkalosis.

This binary buffer model with a buffer strenth as high as 44 slykes, however, did not actually mirror the changes which would occur in human blood during hypothermia. The $\Delta pH/^\circ C$, for example, was only .012 whereas the Rosenthal factor for blood is .0147 and the $\Delta pH/^\circ C$ in the poiklotherms described by Rahn and Reeves [2] was .016. In the blood of all vertebrates, $\Delta pH/^\circ C$ is different in different areas of the temperature range. Between 7 and 17° C it is .017; from 17°–27° it is .0158; and between 27° and 37° it is .014. Moreover, it will be significantly affected by dilution of the blood to lower hematocrit levels.

In modern cardiopulmonary bypass with hypothermia (H-CPBP) the blood of the patient is diluted for rheological reasons to an hematocrit level of 20 to 30, from a normal value of about 40. This step is critical in lowering the incidence of erythrocyte agglutination and sludging and of deviations in the clotting mechanisms during and after perfusion. Much more complete capillary bed perfusion is achieved, with better tissue metabolism during perfusion and with fewer complications relating to blood clotting in the post-operative period. For these reasons, priming the pump with hemoglobin and protein free saline solutions to a volume which, when mixed by the pump with the patient's blood volume, will result in a perfusion fluid with an hemotocrit of 20–25.[2]

Reeves has stated, 'any experimental manipulation which alters plasma protein concentration or hemoglobin levels has a direct effect on the measured pH temperature coefficient $(\Delta pH/^\circ C)$' [4]. A binary buffer model which contains 20–30 mM/l of imidizole with 25 mM/l $NaHCO_3$ was directly applicable to the measured responses in pH and P_{CO_2} of frog blood and plasma subjected to

2. Common solutions combine a commercial extracellular salt solution buffered to pH 7.4 (about 2 liters), 25 mM $NaHCO_3$, with or without mannitol or dextrose (± 200 mM 10% D).

cooling. Dog plasma responded in similar fashion [4]. Similarly, human blood with normal plasma protein is thought to contain approximately 30 mM/l of imidizole. This concentration causes the non-bicarbonate buffer strength of normal blood to approximate 28 slykes. This buffering capacity is divided evenly between the erythrocytes (hemoglobin) and plasma proteins. The former provides 20 slykes; plasma is credited with 8 slykes. Both components have similar pH temperature coefficients.

In a attempt to develop a graph which might serve as a nomogram for respiratory acid-base changes during current H-CPBP procedures, Kindig presented an analysis [5] which showed that when human blood undergoes erythrocyte dilution by 50% to an hemotocrit of 20, associated with similar plasma dilution, the buffer strength falls about 33%. Thus, whole blood with a buffer strength of 28, diluted to an hematocrit of 20, now has a buffer strength of 20 slykes.

This dilution so affects the pH temperature coefficient that it becomes stable at .016. This coefficient places the pH isopleths in a precisely horizontal position on a log P_{CO_2}-T diagram. Thus on such a diagram pH remains constant at any P_{CO_2} concentration throughout the temperature range of 17° to 37° C. Thus it is a remarkable coincidence that current practice for H-CPBP calls for dilution of the blood to an hemotocrit level of about 20, which results in a buffer strength of 20 slykes, a value at which pH and log P_{CO_2} lines charted versus temperature remain perfectly horizontal. With a $\Delta pH/°C$ of .016 this graph describes the acid-base parameters of any point when T_{CO_2} remains constant or is altered by respiration, for the temperature range 17° to 37° C, a range experienced by man undergoing H-CPBP in 1984. Figure 1 is such a diagram. It could easily be used by perfusionists as a nomogram for the management of H-CPBP.

In the interpretation of this diagram the reader must recognize that as a patient cools, his acid-base status will follow some course from right to left starting on the vertical 37° C line or near it, then proceeding left towards the 17° C line. A point with commonly accepted normal values for pH and P_{CO_2} was adopted as the point of beginning. All patients, therefore, are illustrated as entering the graph at point A. The solid lines pointing left illustrate the locus of the pH and P_{CO_2} values which will be found when three specific acid-base management strategies are successfully achieved.

Consider line AD first; this is the line of biologic neutrality determined by the near identity of the change due to falling temperatures in the dissociation constant of water (pKw) and the dissociation constant of imidizole (pKIm). Because of these pK changes, as the body cools the pH will steadily rise while the P_{CO_2} steadily falls, provided that T_{CO_2} remains constant. Note that pH, the negative log of the hydrogen ion concentration, marked on the left hand ordinate scale, is largest at the top of the scale whereas log P_{CO_2}, indicated on the right hand ordinate scale, is smallest at the top of the scale. The two functions are intimately related and can simultaneously follow the same line on the graph. Thus, if the $\dot{V}g/\dot{V}b$ ratio of the perfusion is properly adjusted to achieve this strategy, the in

84

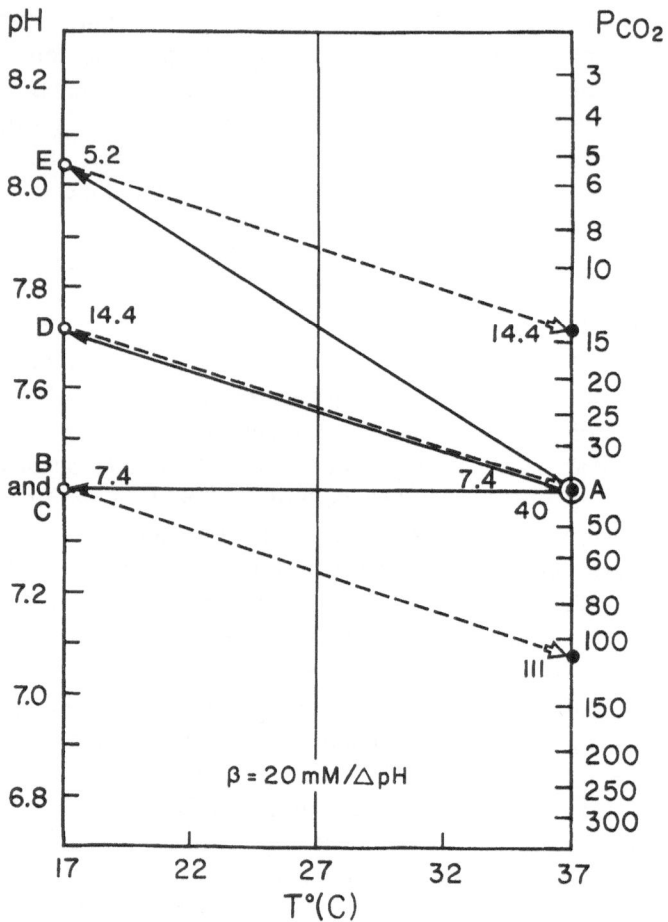

Fig. 1. Graphic depiction of pH, P_{CO_2}, and temperature relationships when the patient's blood has been diluted to a hematocrit of 20%, based on calculations made by Kindig [97]. Buffer strength is now 20 slykes. $\Delta pH/°C$ with this dilution is .016. The pH isopleths are horizontal. The variable is change in T_{CO_2} due to ventilation. This chart approximates common current experience in the operating room. Reproduced by permission of Surgery, Gynecology, and Obstetrics, Chicago, Ill., U.S.A.

vivo values of pH and P_{CO_2} will fall on line AD; the pH at 27° is 7.56 and at 17° is 7.72. Corresponding values for P_{CO_2} are 26 and 14.4, respectively.

Line AD represents particularly the acid-base vs. temperature when T_{CO_2} remains constant. It represents the strategy which Reeves called 'alphastat' [3]. It is this biologically neutral condition which maintains a stable OH^-/H^+ ratio, a constant alpha-imidazole, and a constant protein charge state, thus preserving protein functions which depend on charge state (especially enzyme function). The dashed line leading left to right which is shown close to and parallel to line AD represents the pH and P_{CO_2} values which would occur in a blood sample in a syringe or in the chamber of a blood gas analyzer as it is being warmed from the temperature at which it was drawn to 37° C, the temperature at which the analyzer reads and reports the sample values. Thus the reader should understand that all the dashed lines running from left to right represent the changes which occur in pH and P_{CO_2} when a sample of blood is warmed. These changes, of course, because they occur in a sealed environment, must parallel the biological line AD where T_{CO_2} remains absolutely constant. Thus, all the meter readings illustrated in the graph lie on the 37° vertical line, and are represented by solid circles.

Line AD has the characteristics of a biologic absolute. In all aqueous buffer systems containing imidazole and bicarbonate, no matter in what concentrations, the line represents biologic neutrality. All points on the graph below this line at any temperature represent a state of acidosis. Any point above the line depicts an acid-base state of alkalosis. The further above or below AD the greater the variance from biologic neutrality.

Strategy AB-C depicts the most common currently sought acid-base management strategy. It is achieved by adding CO_2 to the respiratory gas mixture. That this strategy is based on erroneous opinion and ill-advised objectives is the burden of this report. To maintain a constant in vivo pH of 7.4 and P_{CO_2} of 40 torr is to explore the depths of respiratory acidosis. There is no question that this is harmful, especially to the patient's heart (vide infra). At 17° the 'uncorrected' meter readings will be pH 7.08 and P_{CO_2} 111. This is a degree of respiratory acidosis severe enough to threaten the successful outcome of the operation if it is prolonged.

Strategy AE illustrates an attempt at significant respiratory alkalosis achieved by hyperventilation. The open circle at E represents successful achievement of this strategy at 17° C. At this point the in vivo pH is 8.2 and P_{CO_2} is only 5.2 torr. The warming blood sample following the dashed line left to right will lead to a 37° meter reading of pH 7.72 and P_{CO_2} 14.4. This is genuine alkalosis.

Figure 1, it must be noted, represents only patients who have had their blood diluted with a non-protein priming solution. Since the buffer strength of the perfusion fluid has been reduced by a third of that contained in whole blood, it should not be concluded, just because this is common practice, that the technique is ideal. It surely would be possible to retain the full buffering strength of whole blood in spite of dilution if the diluting fluid contained significant non-bicarbonate buffer strength. If a priming fluid could be produced at reasonable economic cost which contained sufficient imidazole to achieve a resultant perfusion solution with a buffer strength of at least 28, (equivalent to whole blood) it would appear desirable to do so.

Thus one could enjoy the undoubted advantages of dilution perfusion, but also maintain the full buffering capacity of whole blood to support good acid-base balance during the hypothermia. The $\Delta pH/° C$ would now increase to .0147, a return to the biochemical potentials inherent in the Rosenthal factor. If such a priming fluid were to be developed, a new diagrammatic nomogram would need to be derived.

Ventilation during surface cooling

Surface cooling was the modality almost universally adopted in the 1950's and early 1960's [6, 7, 8] for the clinical application of hypothermia to heart surgery. It was also utilized primarily in infants to achieve deep hypothermia for the repair of congenital cardiac defects [9, 10, 11, 12, 13]. With the steadily increasing reliability of pump-oxygenator systems and the availability of highly efficient heat exchangers, surface cooling has been almost entirely abandoned in the United States as well as in Europe and in the Far East. Thus, a detailed analysis of the acid-base consequences of various ventilatory techniques to be used by the anesthesiologist before and after cardio-pulmonary bypass is now only occasionally pertinent to the management of gas exchange during hypothermia. During the operative period when ventilation of the lungs is the responsibility of the anesthesiologist, the patient's temperature is within a very few degrees of normal. Not until the perfusionist begins perfusion is hypothermia initiated. However, it seems obvious that a cooperative plan of management by the anesthesiologist and perfusionist will serve the needs of the patient best.

In terms of the management strategies of acid-base during the hypothermia outlined above, it is to be emphasized that these are based entirely on respiratory changes in T_{CO_2} in relationship to temperature. If tissue oxygenation by perfusion is adequate, metabolic acidosis due to hypoxia is unlikely to be superimposed. It would be well for the anesthesiologist to adopt a pulmonary ventilatory program appropriate to the strategy which the perfusionist will adopt when hypothermia is being induced. The rate of CO_2 elimination must be matched in the steady state to the rate of metabolic CO_2 production in a purposeful fashion to achieve each of the strategies.

A beginning approximation of total ventilatory requirements can be made by consideration of the alveolar air equation for CO_2. In the absence of any added CO_2 to the gas mixture this equation is:

$$\dot{V}a = b(T)\dot{V} CO_2/PaCO_2 \text{ where}$$

b(T) relates standard temperature-pressure-dry to body temperature-barometric pressure-saturated gas volumes (b(37°) = .863); $\dot{V}CO_2$ describes the metabolic rate (CO_2 production); and $PaCO_2$ represents the rate of removal of CO_2 by alvealor ventilation.

In this equation if alveolar P_{CO_2} is equal to pulmonary artery P_{CO_2} no alveolar gradient for CO_2 would be present. In normal healthy man at 37° this is assumed to be the case. The question is, does hypothermia affect the CO_2 gradient?

This question was briefly reviewed by Blair [14]; and in 1948, Otis and Jude [15] found no significant interference with transfer of either O_2 or CO_2 at 16° C. Severinghaus and his co-workers found no alteration in total compliance, alveolar dead space, or A-a CO_2 gradients [16, 17]. Total compliance and resistance are unchanged at 29° C in man [18]. Thus, based on these few studies, the opinion can be expressed that hypothermia does not cause significant alteration in any factors except b(T) in the alveolar equation, and this change is relatively small.

If this equation is applied to a patient with the commonly accepted Q_{10} [19] of 2.08 which corresponds to a 7% per degree change in metabolism, the metabolic rate at 17° C is 23% of its 37° value. Using the starting (37°) and ending (17°) P_{CO_2}'s from Fig. 1, we find the following ventilatory requirements at 17° as a percentage of the 37° ventilation needed to achieve the three strategies:

AB-C (constant pH and P_{CO_2})	$.23 \div 40/40 = .23$ (23%)
AD (constant T_{CO_2})	$.23 \div 14.4/40 = .64$ (64%)
AE (lowered T_{CO_2})	$.23 \div 5.2/40 = 1.77$ (177%)

The sharply reduced alveolar ventilation requirement in the acidotic AB-C is impractical because sufficient oxygen might not be delivered. This creates the requirement that CO_2 be added to the inspired gas.

There are two important variables that render this analysis theoretical and subject to doubt. The first is the use for the cardiac patient of the commonly accepted Q_{10} of 2.08, a 7% per degree decrease in $\dot{V}CO_2$. The second is that the alveolar equation does not recognize the changes in respiratory tree anatomical and physiological dynamics. The anesthesiologist is interested in total ventilation ($\dot{V}E/\dot{V}O_2$), not merely alveolar ventilation. These two factors will be discussed in order.

Human Q_{10} values during hypothermia

Measurement of human Q_{10} values during H-CPBP has varied considerably. For example, Prakash et al. [20] found in infants a Q_{10} close to 1.72, a $\Delta\dot{V}O_2$ of 5.3% per degree Celsius. Nealon and Gosin [21] reported $\dot{V}O_2$ in adults was 50% at 28° C, which computes to $\Delta\dot{V}O_2$ of 6.7% per ° C. Reitz and Ream [22] propose 7.3%/° C, and Q_{10} of 2.13. And Fox et al. [23], in very careful studies, reported $\Delta\dot{V}O_2$ to be 8.44, a Q_{10} of 2.4.

That this variable could tremendously influence the proper ventilatory rate is illustrated in Table 1, which is based on the alveolar gas exchange equation and assumes no change in the $PACO_2$–$PaCO_2$ gradient with cooling.

Table 1 shows the effect that Q_{10} would have on the ventilation volume necessary to achieve the alpha-stat strategy AD as the patient's temperature falls to 17° during surface cooling. The so-called 'normal' is based upon the $\Delta P_{CO_2}/° C$ which is seen in human blood subjected to cooling and rewarming when T_{CO_2} is held constant. The ratio of in vivo $P_{CO_2}/37P_{CO_2}$ is always .36. This corresponds to a 5% reduction in P_{CO_2} per ° C $[(1-.05)^{20} = .36]$. In Fig. 1, this is the description of $P_{CO_2}/° C$ which fits the alpha-stat line AD. Since this is the line characterized by constant T_{CO_2}, by definition $\dot{V}CO_2 = PaCO_2$; and a 5% change in $\dot{V}CO_2$ would require 'normal' ventilation to achieve equilibrium where T_{CO_2} remains constant.

Table 1. Surface cooling: Ventilation (minute volume) required to maintain biological neutrality (assuming no change in pulmonary efficiency)

Q_{10}	$\Delta VCO_2/° C$	Ventilation
1.67	5%	Normal
1.72 (20)	5.3%	94% of Normal
2.03 (21)	6.7%	67%
2.08 (19)	7%	64%
2.13 (22)	7.3%	61%
2.4 (23)	8.4%	48%

$\dot{V}CO_2/° C = 5\%$ translates to a Q_{10} of 1.67, where $\dot{V}CO_2 = \dot{V}O_2$.

Inspection of Table 1 suggests that the greater the Q_{10} the less the ventilation required to achieve alpha-stat conditions as the patient cools.

However, this analysis would be completely flawed if one assumption were unwarranted, namely, that there is a specific constant Q_{10} (or $\dot{V}CO_2$) for any patient during cooling, and that there is a direct relationship between metabolic rate and body temperature. In fact, the change in $\dot{V}CO_2$ as temperature falls is subject to so many variables that a precise graph of $\dot{V}CO_2$ expressed as a per cent of normal vis-a-vis temperature cannot be drawn with present data; indeed, it seems unlikely that such a relationship actually exists, except in a general sense. The different components of metabolic rate change differently with cooling (RQ is variable); the endocrine effects on metabolism will vary with changing psychic states and with anesthesia; different organs have different Q_{10}'s and are at different temperatures (large internal thermal gradients exist during cooling and rewarming); oxygen consumption will change with various pump flow rates at hypothermic temperatures; and $\dot{V}CO_2$ will also change with oxyhemoglobin dissociation curves under the influence of pH and P_{CO_2} (see [24] for discussion). One can be sure that under the conditions of whole body cooling and rewarming in man, no single $\dot{V}CO_2$ exists throughout the body and no single temperature represents 'body temperature' (see below). These conditions may exist in poikilo-therms undergoing very gradual thermal change, but they do not exist in humans during clinical hypothermia.

Total ventilation ($\dot{V}_E$) vs. alveolar ventilation ($\dot{V}a$)

Rahn and Reeves [25] have stated that during human hypothermia induced by surface cooling maintenance of a constant ventilatory minute volume is necessary to keep T_{CO_2} constant and thus to achieve alphastat biologic neutrality throughout. This opinion is based on analogy with the behavior of poikilotherms. If Prakash's Q_{10} of 1.72 [20] were reasonably accurate, normal ventilation would fall only a little to the alkaline side of alphastat on the basis of the alveolar equation alone. However, if the commonly accepted Q_{10} of 2.08 more closely approximates a realistic average, then as we have seen in Table 1, only 64% of normal alveolar ventilation would be appropriate to maintain alphastat. Under the latter conditions, the poikiltherms observed by Rahn and Reeves [25, 26] must have experienced significant decrease in overall ventilatory efficiency with cooling, so that steady ventilation would not become severe hyperventilation with the lowering of $\dot{V}CO_2$ associated with falling temperature. To achieve this status of constant T_{CO_2} total ventilation must decrease during a fall in body temperature, i.e., the ratio $\dot{V}E/\dot{V}CO_2$ must rise significantly, *unless ventilatory efficiency* is equally decreased.

That this situation exists in fact with oxygen uptake in the *Pseudomys florinda* has been shown by White [27]. In these animals the $\dot{V}E/\dot{V}O_2$ ratio has increased from 20 at 37° to 50 at 17°. Since the turtle is known to have preserved alphastat acid-base status, the total CO_2 did not change. Thus, in this species, as body temperature fell, because of increasing inefficiency of O_2 and CO_2 pulmonary exchange, a constant 37° ventilatory volume maintained total CO_2 constant, despite decreasing metabolic rate throughout the temperature range of 37° C to 17° C.

Whether the human responds similarly to hypothermia is not fully known, Severinghaus and Larson [17], however, reported bronchodilation and an increase in anatomic dead space of 50%, which might be a change of sufficient magnitude to significantly decrease the volume of alveolar ventilation. The relationship between total exchange and alveolar exchange is commonly thought to be $\dot{V}E = \dot{V}a$ + (respiratory frequency × dead space). At 20° C in man, these computations would suggest VE = Va+ 300 ml air per minute at a frequency of 15. This amounts to only a 10–15% increase in 37° $\dot{V}E$ (original). There may also be a circulatory problem associated with posture. Rahn *et al.* [28] have demonstrated changes in the ventilation perfusion ratios of upper and lower lung lobes with changes in posture.

At the present time, therefore, in the absence of any reliable relationship in man between metabolic rate and temperature which might make Q_{10} either measurable or meaningful, the absence of a realistic 'body temperature' as currently measured, and the lack of solid information concerning respiratory efficiency during hypothermia, an opinion as to the ventilatory volume necessary to achieve alphastat or low T_{CO_2} alkalosis in the management of human H-CPBP is at best an educated guess.

It may well be wise to accept the advice of Rahn and of Prakash and maintain normothermic ventilation, which will probably result in either alphastat or mild alkalosis. Progress can be closely monitored by blood-gas determinations, and appropriate gas exchange modifications made. Maintenance of a 37 pH of 7.4 and 37 P_{CO_2} of 40 torr should be the minimum absolute requirement.

However, as mentioned above the entire subject of ventilation vis-a-vis temperature is little related to the almost universal current practice of inducing and maintaining hypothermia by perfusion. Hypothermia in modern cardiac surgery is machine-induced, and during hypothermia acid-base balance is regulated by in artificial 'lung' not subject to the functional aberrations of the living lung. The gas-blood flow ratio ($\dot{V}_g/\dot{V}_b$) as adjusted by the perfusionist will determine acid-base status. These will be constrained by the parameters of the weight and age of the patient, the volume of return flow available to recycle in the P-O, the specific gas exchange characteristics of the oxygenator (bubble, disc, screen or membrane), the venous P_{CO_2}, and blood gas monitoring of arterial and venous blood. The accumulated experience of the perfusionist will provide a proximate pattern with which to begin. Monitoring is then the key. It would help if at the time perfusion cooling begins, the patient were in a state of respiratory alkalosis achieved by the anesthesiologist by moderate hyperventilation. The perfusionist would best be served if only an instrument were available at the venous return port of the oxygenator which would yield continuous on-line measurements of pH, P_{CO_2}, P_{O_2}, and temperature. Until such refinements are available, the first important blood sample should be drawn about 15 minutes before perfusion will probably begin. The results will be posted in the OR just in time to give the perfusionist an idea of the acid-base status of the patient at the onset of his perfusion. A sample 10 minutes later will start a series of measurements to monitor success in achieving the acid-base strategy which has been elected for that patient. The use of Fig. 1 as a nomogram might be very helpful.

CO₂ and the heart

In the early application of hypothermia to open heart surgery, extensive experience in the experimental laboratory with dogs led Swan *et al.* [7] to adapt and to recommend the use of vigorous hyperventilation throughout the course of clinical hypothermia. A rectal temperature of 28–30° was sought. At this level of hypothermia 37 pH was 7.56 ± .9. This recommendation was made because this degree of respiratory alkalosis apparently stabilized the rhythm of the cold heart. Ventricular fibrillation, the early bête noire of canine hypothermia, was almost entirely eliminated, and electric shock defibrillation, when needed, became effective and reliable. This respiratory strategy was widely adopted for surface cooling without perfusion in the middle and late 1950's [6]. The Japanese used this technique [9, 10, 13] to explore surface-induced deep hypothermia with prolonged circulatory arrest. Respiratory alkalosis was later fully endorsed by Mohri and his group at Seattle in an extensive experience with surface-induced deep hypothermia for the correction of congenital cardiac defects in infants [11, 12, 30, 31]. Strong experimental evidence has documented a favorable effect of both respiratory and metabolic alkalosis on cardiac contractility and more importantly on the recovery of contractility after a period of prolonged ischemia at normothermia.

That an alkalosis also has a beneficial effect upon circulatory dynamics at deep hypothermic temperatures was indicated by the experimental studies of Wang and Katz [32] who found a decrease in myocardial contractile force with acidosis induced by coronary infusion of DMO and Na_2CO_3. Ebert *et al.* [33] showed that during hypothermia in dogs to 12° C associated with 30 minutes of aortic occlusion, if the perfusate were made alkaline (pH 7.6) by the addition of $NaHCO_3$, post-occlusion myocardial contractility was markedly improved compared to controls or ones given dilute HCl.

That severe acidosis occurs during myocardial ischemia even if the heart is protected by topical cooling to 16° C was documented by Follette *et al.* [34]. In their animals coronary sinus pH fell at an ever-increasing rate to 6.8 during one hour of aortic occlusion. These data are graphed in Fig. 2.

They also clearly showed that the pH of the blood used to reperfuse after one hour of hypothermic aortic occlusion had a critical effect on the return of myocardial contractility toward control values as measured at 30 minutes. The optimal pH level for reperfusion was 7.7–7.9. This striking phenomenon is illustrated in Fig. 3.

McConnell *et al.* in 1975 [35] manipulated blood pH by hyperventilation and injecting $NaHCO_3$. Their dogs were cooled to 28° C with CPBP. When the pH (corrected for temperature) was elevated to 7.72 and compared to those main-

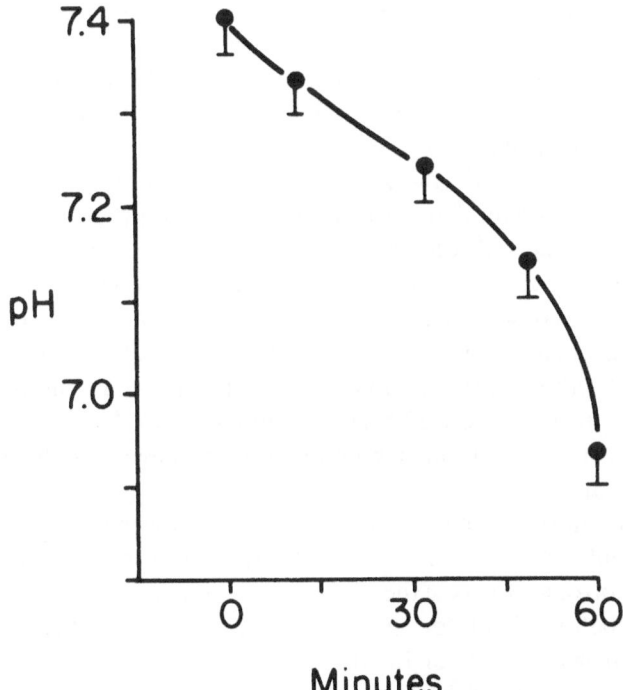

Fig. 2. Coronary sinus blood pH during one hour of myocardial ischemia at 16° C. Reproduced as modified with permission of C.V. Mosby, St. Louis, Mo., U.S.A.

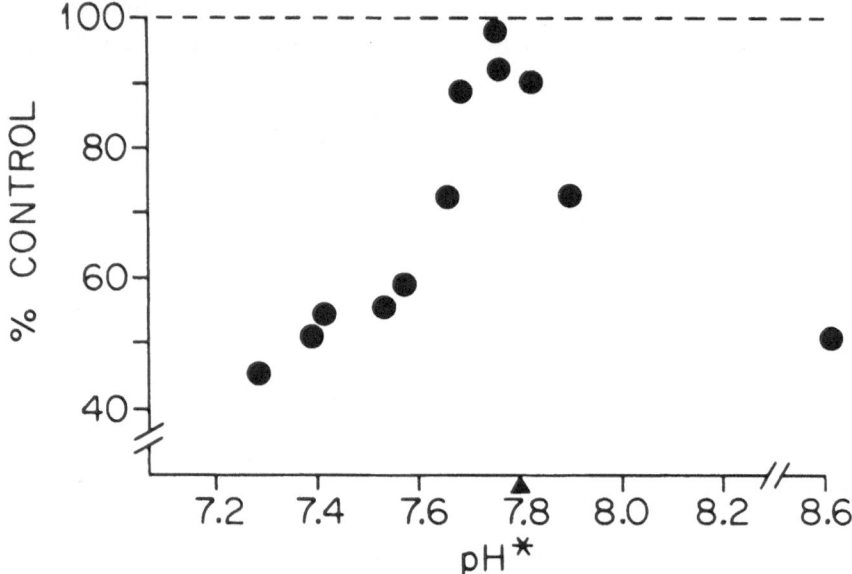

Fig. 3. Left ventricular performance (intra-ventricular balloon dp/dt values) 30 minutes after one hour of ischemic arrest at 16° C compared to pre-arrest values when initial reperfusate at 30° C was modified from pH 7.3 to pH 8.6. The clearcut superiority of reperfusion at pH 7.8 is evident [34]. Reproduced as modified with permission of C.V. Mosby, St. Louis, Mo., U.S.A.

tained at 7.4 a definite increase in total left ventricular coronary blood flow, particularly in the subendocardial region was seen. This was accompanied by an increase in left ventricular performance.

Recently, in an important (but frequently confusing) report Becker *et al.* [36] presented convincing data that with surface cooling of puppies subendorcardial blood flow and cardiac index fell less with marked respiratory alkalosis (pH 8.1) than with maintenance of pH of 7.4 at 37° C, and moreover, lactacidemia was avoided, and excess base remained normal during post-arrest perfusion rewarming. Most striking of all, however, was the rapid return of left ventricular function toward normal with hyperventilation in contrast to the lingering suppression of left ventricular function where 37 pH was maintained at 7.4. The relative position of these studies to those of Rahn in poikilotherms is shown, together with the data of McConnell, in Fig. 4.

Thus, in summarizing the studies on alkalosis, the strength of myocardial contraction is enhanced at a pH of 7.7 to 8.1 at temperatures below 30°. Moreover, the negative inotropic effects of the acidosis of ischemia are partially prevented by alkalinization before circulatory occlusion, and significantly benefited by initial alkaline reperfusion at a pH of 7.8 at 30° C.

Nonetheless, throughout the recent use of hypothermia for open-heart surgery there have been those who recommended respiratory acidosis. It has been suggested that ventricular fibrillation was a result of myocardial hypoxia. How-

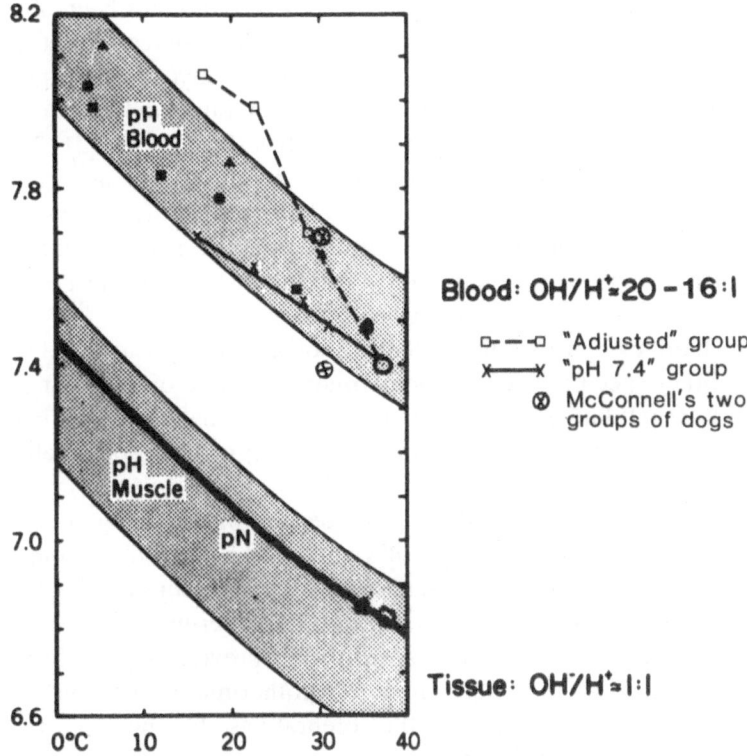

Fig. 4. Data from McConnell *et al.* [35] and Becker *et al.* [36] are superimposed on a typical diagram modified from Rahn. Alpha-stat management (Strategy AD) is identical to 'pH 7.4' group. The severe alkalosis of Becker's 'adjusted pH' puppies relative to Rahn's poikilotherms is evident. Reproduced by permission of Surgery, Gynecology, and Obstetrics, Chicago, Ill., U.S.A.

ever, this conception has been proven wrong in several ways. At colder temperatures the much diminished metabolic needs would be adequately met by oxygen transported in solution, if flow is adequate. That this is indeed the case was demonstrated independently by Gollan [37, 38] and by Boerema *et al.* [39]. Below 12° C, more oxygen is presented by perfusion to the heart dissolved in plasma than the measured myocardial consumption requires. In the Alaskan ice fish [40] at −2° C the entire animal can be fully oxygenated without benefit of any hemoglobin. In Boerema's colorful phraseology, there is 'life without blood'. Hypoxia, since it is rarely present in simple deep hypothermia without aortic cross-clamping, is not the cause of cardiac irritability.

If intermittent ischemia is superimposed, however, intermittent coronary perfusion of the cold arrested myocardium during aortic cross-clamping can maintain myocardial integrity and meet its energy requirements, but at least a 10% hematocrit blood solution is required [41]. The importance of these data will be apparent in subsequent discussion of cardiopreservation.

That systemic acidosis reduces myocardial contractility has been abundantly documented during the last 100 years. Moreover, the progressive extra-cellular acidosis of ischemia is the specific cause of loss of myocardial function and eventual cellular death. So much data have been generated to this effect that only a partial listing of the references is possible in this short paper. [21, 35, 37, 38, 42–55]. At some point the functional loss of the acidotic cell becomes irreversible. Since the point of irreversibility in the course of progressive myocardial acidosis is clearly determinant of the permissible duration of aortic clamping in adult heart surgery, further steps to prevent it or reverse it should be the subject of increased interest to surgical teams. This is discussed further below.

Despite all this evidence of the cardiac risks of respiratory acidosis, the effect of CO_2 upon other specific vascular compartments became of overriding concern during the 1960's. It had been shown in 1928 [56] in animals, and later in man [57, 58] that an increase in blood CO_2 exerts a vasodilating effect on cerebral blood vessels.

In 1954, Parkins *et al.* [59] had described serious brain damage in dogs when cerebral temperature was lower than 14° C; and Bjork and Hultquist in 1962 [60] published a chilling paper which described focal brain lesions leading to death in five children undergoing profound perfusion hypothermia. These reports and others [61, 62] rightfully caused widespread critical review of hypothermic techniques. Concern about the effect of deep hypothermia on the central nervous system led to increasing interest in the cerebral vasodilating capacity of CO_2. Because of the suspected risk to the brain of perfusion, and because of the use of prolonged total circulatory arrest, it was deemed advisable to add CO_2 to the anesthetic and oxygenator gases to 'help cool the brain' [63] and to provide maximum pre-occlusion oxidation.

Indeed, this practice of inducing respiratory acidosis by adding CO_2 to the anesthetic inspired gas and to the oxygenator gas flow became almost universally adopted by cardio-pulmonary bypass teams across the United States [6, 22, 64, 65]. Only recently, a few groups particularly aware of the bad effects of acidosis on myocardial function have begun to question the wisdom of this practice [20, 23, 29, 66].

In evaluating this question, it is important to identify precisely which organs or systems are specifically in jeopardy as hypothermia deepens, pump times become more and more prolonged, and the period of aortic crossclamping or total circulatory arrest stretches to unexpected lengths. Under present circumstances it can be agreed that the two organs at most risk are the heart and the brain.

Current CPBP has divided itself into two quite distinct techniques depending on the patient's age and weight. Infants undergo quite a different experience than children or adults. The usual cut-off weight is 10 kg. These two methods will be examined in particular relationship to the constraints enforced by the separate tolerances of the heart and the brain (Fig. 5).

For adults, CPBP is the primary modality for total body life support; hypother-

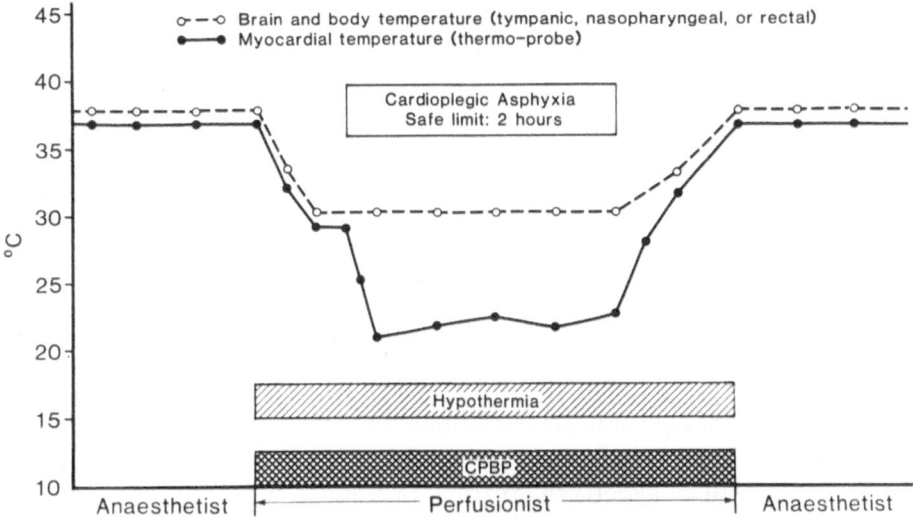

Fig. 5. The relationship of brain and body temperature to myocardial temperature during the course of adult cardiopulmonary bypass. During aortic cross-clamping, only the heart is ischemic. Reproduced by permission of Surgery, Gynecology, and Obstetrics, Chicago, Ill., U.S.A.

mia of moderate degree, i.e., 26°–30° C, is used as an adjunct to diminish the perfusion volume needed to maintain body oxygen levels. Oxygen demand has fallen at least 50% at these levels. During the operation, the isolated heart will undergo additional local hypothermia to 16°–20° C, while total body perfusion continues at the 26°–30° C level. Since hypothermia is perfusion-induced the perfusionist is in charge of the welfare of the patient throughout the hypothermic experience. Inasmusch as the heart is 90% isolated from perfusion and its deep hypothermia is controlled by the surgeon, the protection of the myocardium during aortic crossclamping becomes the responsibility of the surgeon. Meanwhile, however, throughout the operation until the patient is fully rewarmed, the brain and the rest of the body are being perfused by the perfusionist. The brain, therefore, is not at great risk even were the operation to last for 4 or 5 hours. These considerations are emphasized in Table 2.

For infants and younger children up to about 10 kg, profound hypothermia to a TB of 12°–16° is sought either by surface cooling, by CPBP, or a combination of both. At an appropriate moment, illustrated in Fig. 6, total circulatory arrest is induced and continued without interruption while surgery proceeds. Based on early experiences, sixty minutes of CA has been thought to be safe [33]. But recent studies throw grave doubt on this figure. Indeed, after about 40 minutes progressive brain damage with cerebral functional loss begins to occur (vide infra). When cardiac repair is complete, the patient is warmed with perfusion. The perfusionist is in charge of both hypothermia and CPBP through the operation. As is emphasized in Table 3, since the brain is the more sensitive to ischemia,

Table 2. Adult and childhood CPBP with general hypothermia and aortic cross clamping

1. Pump-oxygenator used primarily for total body respiration. Heat exchange a secondary function.
2. Moderate general hypothermia an adjunct to perfusion; local myocardial cooling.
3. Brain and heart undergo different hypothermic experiences.
   a. Brain: Moderate hypothermia; continuous oxygenation.
   b. Heart: Profound hypothermia; prolonged asphyxia.
4. Non-coronary collateral flow 'washes out' cardioplegic solution during aortic cross-clamping.
5. Perfusionist in charge of patient's welfare throughout hypothermia.
6. Surgeon responsible for myocardial damage during ischemia: Temperature control; cardio-preservation solution.
7. Ischemic threat to cardiac function the overriding constraint on aortic cross-clamping.

it becomes the limiting parameter of the duration of the procedure. If circulatory arrest is stretched too far, the heart and brain become rivals as threats to survival.

Only 6 to 8% of all hypothermic cardiac operations with circulatory occlusion or arrest are in infant patients. Of these approximately 65% can be completed in less than 50 minutes. The longer, more complex and time consuming operations comprise the arena wherein careful consideration of acid-base management and careful timing will spell the difference between low-risk, complication-free recovery and a high risk of serious cardiac and cerebral morbidity.

CO_2 and the brain

Since the rationale for adding CO_2 to the respiratory gas particularly in infants

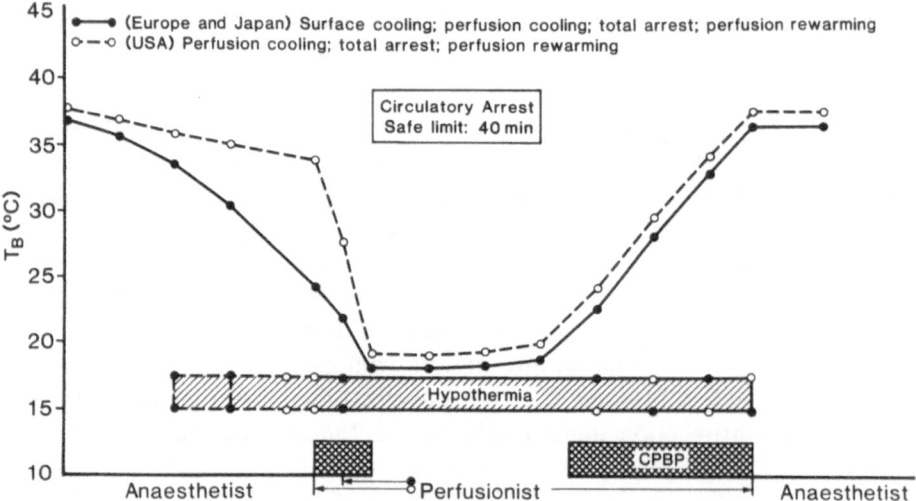

Fig. 6. During infant CPBP using deep hypothermia, all the tissues suffer an equal period of ischemia. Reproduced by permission of Surgery, Gynecology, and Obstetrics, Chicago, Ill., U.S.A.

Table 3. Infant CPBP with profound hypothermia and total circulatory arrest

1. Pump oxygenator used primarily as heat exchanger.
2. Profound total-body hypothermia the basic cardio-surgical modality.
3. Heart and brain undergo identical ischemic hypothermic experiences.
4. No 'washout' of cardioplegic solution during cardiac operation.
5. Perfusionist is in charge of both CPBP and hypothermia throughout.
6. Tolerance of cold brain to ischemia is overriding constraint on circulatory arrest.

was to achieve cerebral vascular dilation and hopefully therefore to protect the brain, it would be very useful to have some late follow-up studies, both with and without the added CO_2. No such study can be found in the literature. However, several studies of cerebral metabolism and blood flow at various temperatures and CO_2 tensions are available.

In one careful study in the dog [67], respiratory alkalosis did decrease blood flow, but this did not impair the hypothermic cerebral metabolism. Exactly similar conclusions were drawn by Hagerdal *et al.* [68] and Carlson *et al.* [69] in studies in the rat.

Becker *et al.* [36] found in puppies that cardiac index and blood pressure remained higher during surface cooling with hyperventilation, and cerebral blood flow did not fall as much as in animals respired to maintain P_{CO_2} at 35 torr. Moreover, Fox *et al.* [23] have shown that during CPBP with decreasing flow rates the proportion of cerebral to total body flow actually increases even without CO_2, so that there is a preferential blood flow to the brain at low flow rates.

Thus, during CPBP at 20° C conducted using alpha-stat strategy AD, any flow rate adequate to meet total body oxygen demand for aerobic metabolism will automatically and preferentially result in adequate cerebral oxygenation. Adding CO_2 to improve cerebral flow appears to be unnecessary. In infants the duration of circulatory arrest rather than acid-base considerations will be the key parameter of jeopardy to brain function. Several recent follow-up studies on cerebral function and intellectual development following H-CPBP with cardiac arrest in infants [70, 71, 72] have shown the increasing incidence of damage with increasing duration of circulatory arrest. Lincoln *et al.* [73] flatly declare that circulatory arrest of 60 minutes seriously threatens later intellectual development.

Thus the widespread practice of accepting the known myocardial toxicity of mild and severe acidosis in the belief that the brain would be better protected from ischemia has received no support from experimental studies nor from existing post-operative intelligence evaluations. In short, although CO_2 does dilate cerebral blood vessels, it has not been shown to help cerebral preservation during hypothermic ischemia; the only thing that is currently proven about adding CO_2 to the respiratory gas mixture is that the practice is deleterious to the heart.

Since it appears that duration of circulatory arrest is the critical parameter and since it appears that the 'safe' period actually approximates 40 minutes rather than the 60 previously adopted, reperfusion of the brain at 40 minutes seems obviously desirable. Reperfusion was first recommended by Barrett-Boyes [70] when it became clear to the surgeon that the procedure would become unduly prolonged. A decision could be made at 40 minutes whether or not the heart procedure would be completed within the next 5 minutes. If not, perfusion could be started with or without clamping the aorta. Various technical maneuvers are available either to diminish blood escaping into the open right ventricle or to return it to the pump if it does. The perfusion should continue uninterrupted for five minutes, and should result in prolonging safe operating time for another 30 minutes. The myocardium should again be flushed with a coronary infusion of cardiopreservative solution.

The body temperature

As one peruses the literature on the surgical management of perfusion hypothermia one is struck by the frequency with which the term 'body temperature' is used, often with a considerable degree of confidence, as if indeed a single 'body temperature' existed. But in fact, in human H-CPBP there is no such thing as 'a' body temperature. Even in a very stable environment, different temperatures exist throughout the shell as compared to the core. When the body temperatures are changing rapidly, as during the induction of hypothermia by either surface or perfusion cooling, large thermal differences occur between different organs of the core (as well as the distinction between differences between core and shell). These differences are greater with rapid perfusion cooling than with surface cooling, but nonetheless are always present. The blood flow to the various organs varies under these conditions, so that warm tissues with high metabolic rates may be relatively poorly perfused with cold blood; hypoxic metabolism in these areas may contribute to a general acidosis. Minimizing internal thermal gradients is an important reason for combining surface cooling and rewarming with perfusion as a better modality of inducing hypothermia [8, 20, 74].

This fact emphasizes the tremendous practicality of strategy AD. With this acid-base management internal temperature gradients make no difference since every tissue in the body, no matter what its temperature, will be at biologic neutrality.

Thus, on the basis of the analysis in this review, it is strongly recommended that since CO_2 acidosis is myotoxic, and since CO_2 dilatation of cerebral vessels has not been proven to be of importance for protection of the brain, *no CO_2 should be added to any ventilating gas mixture.* And since management of AD and AE can be easily achieved by using and interpreting the 37 degree meter reading, no temperaure 'correction' should be made.

Cardioplegia

About 10 years ago, attention was again directed toward potecting the heart by eliminating the electromechanical energy requirements and trying to counteract the biochemical lesion of ischemia, especially calcium transport [75–80]. Thus emerged the current era of co-called cardioplegia.

How to achieve instant electromechanical arrest with maximum safety to myocardial function, while at the same time to minimize or delay progressive myocardial damage due to ischemia was the main focus of cardioplegia. Concerning arrest of the heart, potassium solutions were restudied and endorsed [81–85]. Attention was directed toward ameliorating the conglomerates of calcium which are a common sequella of myocardial ischemia. Calcium antagonists such as verapamil and nifedipine also showed promise [86].

All of these various solutions were mildly acidotic and none were deliberately buffered. And all of them received widespread trial in the U.S. and abroad in combination with moderate general hypothermia and deep regional cardiac cooling. Very impressive operative mortality statistics were generated, particularly in operations limited to 1 to $1\frac{1}{2}$ hours. Within this time span, myocardial hypothermia to 15–20° C associated with electro-mechanical arrest repeated intermittently, as necessitated by non-coronary collateral washout of the myocardium, was so successful that a certain complacency on the part of cardiac surgeons emerged. When these time limits were exceeded in more complicated cases, however, operative mortality and the incidence of late myocardiopathies increased dramatically. To many observers, there was still need for improvement.

Brettschneider [87] and Bleese [88] at the 1979 Cardioplegic Workshop in New York began to emphasize repeated cardioplegic myocardial perfusions with *oxygenated* solutions containing suitable buffers, specifically histidine. For the first time since the effect of body temperature on acid-base regulation was presented in the Amberson Lecture by Hermann Rahn in 1975 [26, 89] fell on surgical minds unprepared for such new and tradition shattering concepts of pH and P_{CO_2} during hypothermia, the effect of cold on pK_w, the hydroxyl-hydrogen ratio, the importance of the pK of imidazole, and the whole general idea of alpha-stat acid-base regulation as reviewed by Swan attracted the attention of the cardiac surgeons at that symposium [90].

At the termination of this meeting, it seemed no longer profitable to debate whether hypothermia or cardioplegia was more important in counteracting ischemia [91]. It was recognized that attempts should be made to maintain or restore aerobic metabolism in order to replenish energetic substrates, coupled with all modalities which contribute to non-toxic reversible suppression of metabolic rate, and also coupled with tight control of acid-base state before, during, and after hypothermia and CPBP associated with circulatory arrest. All aspects, in short, of a program designed to prevent ischemic myocardial injury and to treat effectively what does occur would be the goal of a new era dedicated to myocardial preservation. A key aspect of this era, will be the development of ever-improving cardio-preservative solutions.

Cardiopreservation

Studies emerging from the clinic and laboratories of UCLA have in the past defined, and still continue to implement the practice of cardiopreservation. Maloney and Nelson [92] presented the background of the concept in 1975. Cunningham et al. [93], based on the studies of this group, developed a very detailed and comprehensive protocol for the intra-operative protection of myocardial integrity which is a model of modern cardiopreservation. The importance of continuously combating ischemic myocardial acidosis by alkalotic CPBP and coronary perfusion was fully documented in an experimental protocol in puppies by Becker et al. [36]. Markedly improved myocardial and circulatory parameters (including cerabral blood flow) resulted when profound respiratory alkalosis was maintained during immersion hypothermia to 22° C, circulatory arrest for one hour after perfusion cooling to 17° C and induction of cardiac arrest with blood pH 7.8 (cardioplegia), an injection which was repeated upon initiation of reperfusion. The comparison was with a similar protocol where the pH was maintained at 7.4 at 37° C by respiratory control. The experiment closely mimicked the infant clinical procedure. Some deficiency in the presentation of the report caused misinterpretation of the nature of the control group by several commentators [25, 66, 94, 95, 96]; but there was no argument with the superiority of the post-ischemic cardiovascular parameters seen with myocardial protection with profound hypothermia (17°), extreme alkalosis, cardioplegia with blood buffers at pH 7.8, and initial alkalotic reperfusion. This represents an impressive advance into the new era of cardiopreservation.

In October 1983 studies were presented at the Surgical Forum of The American College of Surgeons suggesting the use of oxygen free-radical-scavenging enzymes superoxide dismutase catalase (Casale et al. and Stewart et al.), and the group at UCLA presented evidence of the value of adding the adenine nucleotide precursor glutamine to their blood potassium cardoplegia solution. The addition of Krebs cycle intermediates of nucleotide precursors may prove to be a useful component of cardiopreservative solutions.

In our opinion, a currently acceptable cardiopreservative solution would include the characteristics detailed in Table 4.

For perfusion, one key objective is dilution of the patient's blood to an hemotocrit of 20–25% to avoid sludging, agglutination, and rheological dynamic problems. In so diluting the blood, attention should be paid to preserving the buffer values of the eventual perfusion medium. Thus, the priming solution should be of a sufficient volume, of a suitable hematocrit so that when thoroughly mixed by a pump run with the patient's blood volume (of known hematocrit), the

Table 4. Characteristics of a currently acceptable cardiopreservative solution

1. Fully oxygenated
2. Temperature 4–8° C
3. pH 7.8
4. Binary buffer systems:
   a. 30 mM/l imidazole plus 24 mM/l NaHCO$_3$, or
   b. 20% Hct blood (autologous or bank)
5. Cardioplegic electrolytes:
   a. K$^+$ 20–24 mM/l, Ca^{++} 2 mM/l, Mg^{++} 12 mM/l
6. Energy substrates: 10 mM/l glucose; possibly others
7. Osmolarity 325 mOsm/L; oncotic pressure 35 mmHg.

resultant perfusion fluid will have an hematocrit of 20–25%, and an imidazole-bicarbonate content approximating 25–30 mM/l. The remaining constituents concern iso-osmolarity of normal ions together with some glucose, other energy substrates, and perhaps mannitol to adjust oncotic pressure.

Acid-base balance during hypothermia and CPBP

What, therefore, seems to be the current optimal management of the acid-base aspects of modern H-CPBP operations of the heart?

As regards infant profound hypothermia with total circulatory occlusion, based on the considerations developed above, namely, that CO$_2$ acidosis does not in fact 'protect the brain' and that respiratory alkalosis does in fact preserve myocardial function during circulatory arrest, it is recommended that the anesthetist and perfusionist coordinate their efforts to achieve significant respiratory alkalosis. Strategy AE or a close approximation would appear to be optimal, achieved by respiratory hyperventilation followed by perfusion using a high gas-blood ratio. No CO$_2$ should be added to any gas mixture. The oxygen/compressed air ratio should keep arterial P$_{O_2}$ at a level between 250 and 350, and venous P$_{O_2}$ above 50. At the time of reperfusion the perfusate should be as alkaline as possible.

For the adult, the strategy, which otherwise should be alpha-stat, must also be AE because of the need for cardiopreservation of the ischemic heart. Uncorrected venous pH's 7.7 to 7.9 and P$_{CO_2}$'s of 12 to 20 torr should be sought as the patient cools below 27°. The period in the operation when a highly alkaline perfusion is especially needed is at the moment of unclamping the aorta thereby reperfusing the coronaries. The surgeon should have just finished delivering a cardiopreservative coronary infusion with a solution buffered at pH 7.8. The pump perfusion should continue to combat myocardial acidosis as the patient warms. The perfusionist might anticipate this need by accelerating his gas flow or even adding THAM. At no time should CO$_2$ be added to any gas mixture.

102

Summary

1. Respiratory changes in blood pH, P_{CO_2} and T_{CO_2} in relation to temperature and to buffer strength are graphically presented.
2. Four possible clinical strategies for managing and controlling the acid-base state during H-CPBP are identified and defined.
3. A respiratory acid-base nomogram for blood diluted to an hemotocrit of 20 is presented in graphic form.
4. Modern cardiac operating room procedures resolve themselves into two patterns, infant and adult. In both instances, however, the perfusionist is in control of the management of hypothermia and perfusion-preservation of body and brain.
5. The surgeon must accept responsibility for preservation of the heart.
6. Studies pertinent to the relationship of acid-base state to the functional and structural preservation of the heart and brain during the conditions of cooling and rewarming during hypothermia, prolonged cardiopulmonary bypass, aortic cross-clamping, and total circulatory arrest have been reviewed.
7. There is overwhelming evidence that at any temperature to 15° C myocardial anoxia caused by aortic occlusion or total circulatory arrest results in progressive acidosis which, of itself, is myotoxic.
8. Myocardial ischemia in adults should be prevented and treated by alkaline perfusion cooling and by frequent coronary perfusion of a cardiopreservative solution which is very cold (4–10° C), oxygenated, slightly hyperosmolar, and which contains at least 20% Hct blood (imidazole, rbc, plasma protein colloid), a cardioplegic ionic pattern, and energy substrates.
9. Myocardial acidosis in infants should be prevented and treated by hypothermic alkaline perfusion before circulatory arrest, more frequent use of cardiopreservative solution, and alkaline reperfusion.
10. Evidence is strong that the use of CO_2 gas added to any respiratory mixture is harmful. It increases myocardial acidosis; it does not increase cerebral blood flow during hypothermia.
11. Current periods of infant circulatory arrest are often too prolonged and are resulting in cerebral post-operative deficiency. Temporary resumption of CPBP at 40 minutes should be adopted.
12. The best perfusion acid-base management strategy for infant H-CPBP is significant respiratory alkalosis (Strategy AE).
13. The best acid-base management strategy for adult H-CPBP is likewise significant respiratory alkalosis (AE).
14. The characteristics of an 'ideal' cardiopreservative solution are outlined. Its frequent intermittent use is the responsibility of the surgeon.

References

1. Kindig ML, Filley GF, Swan H: Acid-base balance in clinical profound hypothermia with circulatory arrest: a graphic analysis. Poster presentation, FASEB, 1983.
2. Rahn H, Reeves RB: Patterns in vertebrate acid-base regulation. In: Evolution of Respiratory Processes. A Comparative Approach, Wood SC, Lenfant C (eds). Marcel Dekker Publishers, New York, 1979: 233–235.
3. Reeves RB: An imidazole alphastat hypothesis for vertebrate acid-base regulation; tissue carbon dioxide content and body temperature in bull frogs. Resp Physiol 14: 219–236, 1972.
4. Reeves RB: Temperature-induced changes in blood acid-base status: pH and P_{CO_2} in a binary buffer. J Appl Physiol 40: 752–761, 1976.
5. Kindig NB: Acid-base status of hemoglobin blood buffers during cardiopulmonary bypass. Presented at Conference on physiology and biochemistry of blood gas transport, Canberra, ACT, Australia, September 5, 1983.
6. Michenfelder JD, Terry HR Jr, Daw EG et al.: Induced hypothermia: physiologic effects, indications, and techniques. Surg Clin N Am 45: 889–898, 1965.
7. Swan H, Zeavin I, Holmes JH, Montgomery V: Cessation of circulation in general hypothermia. 1. Physiologic changes and their control. Ann Surg 138: 360–376, 1954.
8. Swan H: Advances in Cardiopulmonary Diseases, Banyai AL, Gordon BL (eds). Year Book Medical Publishers, Chicago, 1962, Vol I: 662–694.
9. Hikasa U, Shirontani H, Satomura K, et al.: Open-heart surgery in infants. Arch Jap Chir 36: 495–504, 1967.
10. Horiuchi T, Koyamado K, Matano I, et al.: Radical operation for ventricular septal defect in infancy. J Thorac Cardiovasc Surg 46: 180–190, 1963.
11. Mohri H, Hessel EA, Nelson RJ, et al.: Use of rheomacrodex and hyperventilation in prolonged circulatory arrest under deep hypothermia induced by surface cooling: method for open heart surgery in infants. Am J Surg 112: 241–250, 1966.
12. Mohri H, Dillard DH, Crawford EW, et al.: Method of surface-induced deep hypothermia for open-heart surgery in infants. J Thorac Cardiovasc Surg 58: 562–570, 1969.
13. Okamoto Y: Clinical studies for open-heart surgery in infants with profound hypothermia. Arch Jap Chir 38: 188–196, 1969.
14. Blair, E: Clinical Hypothermia. McGraw-Hill, New York, 1964: 50–56.
15. Otis AB, Jude J: Effect of body temperature on pulmonary gas exchange. Am J Physiol 188: 355–359, 1957.
16. Seeringhaus JW, Stupfel M, Bradley AF: Alveolar dead space and arterial to end tidal carbon dioxide differences during hypothermia in dog and man. J Appl Physiol 10: 349–355, 1959.
17. Severinghaus JW, Larson CP Jr: Respiration in anesthesia. In: Handbook of Physiology, Section 3, Respiration, Volume II, Fenn WO, Rahn H (eds). The American Physiological Society, Washington, D.C., 1965: 1219–1259.
18. Schezer PH: Effect of hypothermia on compliance and resistance of the lung-thorax system of anesthetized man. J Appl Physiol 13: 53–56, 1958.
19. Van 't Hoff, JH: Etudes sur la dynamique chimique. Muller, Amsterdam, 1884.
20. Prakash O, Jonson B, Bos E, et al.: Cardiorespiratory and metabolic effect of profound hypothermia. Crit Care Med 6: 165–171, 1978.
21. Nealon TF Jr, Gosin S: Hypothermia: Physiologic affects and clinical application. Med Clin N Am 49: 1181–1188, 1965.
22. Reitz BR, Ream AK: Uses of hyothermia in cardiovascular surgey. In: Acute Cardiovascular Management, Anaesthesia and Intensive Care, Ream AK, Fogdall RP (eds). J.B. Lippincott, Philadelphia, 1982: 830–851.
23. Fox LS, Blackstone EH, Kirklin JW, et al.: Relationship of whole body oxygen consumption to perfusion flow rate during hypothermic cardiopulmonary bypass. J Thorac Cardiovasc Surg 83: 239–258, 1982.

104

24. Swan H: Thermoregulation and Bioenergetics. American Elsevier, New York, 1974: 33–45.
25. Rahn H, Reeves RB: Hydrogen ion regulation during hypothermia; from the Amazon to the operating room. In: Applied Physiology in Clinical Respiratory Care, Prakash O (ed). Martinus Nijhoff Publishers, The Hague, 1982: 1–15.
26. Rahn H, Reeves RB, Howell BJ: Hydrogen ion regulation, temperature and evolution (The Amberson Lecture). Am Rev Respir Dis 112: 165–172, 1975.
27. White FN: A comparative physiological approach to hypothermia. Editorial. J Thorac Cardiovasc Surg 82: 821–831, 1981.
28. Rahn H, Sadoul P, Farhi LE, Shapiro J: Distribution of ventilation and perfusion to lobes of the dog's lung. Fed Proc 14: 117, 1955.
29. Blayo MC, Lecompte V, Pocidalo JJ: Control of acid-base status during hypothermia in man. Respir Physiol 42: 287–298, 1980.
30. Rittenhouse EA, Ho CS, Mohri H, et al.: Circulatory dynamics during surface-induced hypothermia and after cardiac arrest for one hour. J Thorac Cardiovasc Surg 50: 359–369, 1971.
31. Wong KC, Mohri H, Dillard DH, et al.: Deep hypothermia and di-ethyl ether anesthesia for open-heart surgery in infants. A clinical report of 8 years' experience. Anesth Anal 53: 765–771, 1974.
32. Wang H, Katz RL: Effects of changes in coronary blood pH on the heart. Circulation Res 17: 114–122, 1965.
33. Ebert PA, Greenfield LJ, Austen WG, et al.: The relationship of blood pH during profound hypothermia on subsequent myocardial function. Surg Gynecol Obstet 114: 357–362, 1962.
34. Follette DM, Fey K, Livesay J, et al.: Studies on myocardial reperfusion injury. I. Favorable modification by adjusting reperfusate pH. Surgery 82: 149–155, 1977.
35. McConnell DH, White FN, Nelson RL, et al.: Importance of alkalosis in maintenance of 'ideal' blood pH during hypothermia. Surg Forum 26: 263–265, 1975.
36. Becker H, Vinton-Johansen J, Buckberg GD, et al.: Myocardial damage caused by keeping pH 7.4 during systemic hypothermia. J Thorac Cardiovasc Surg 82: 810–820, 1981.
37. Gollan F, Hoffman JE, Jones RM: Maintenance of life of dogs below 10° without hemoglobin. Am J Physiol 179: 640–647, 1954.
38. Gollan G: Electrolyte transfer during hypothermia. In: The Physiology of Induced Hypothermia, Dripps RD (ed). Washington NAS-NRC, 1956, Publication 451: 37–41.
39. Boerema I, Wildschut A, Schmidt WJH: Experimental researches into hypothermia as an aid in surgery of the heart. Arch Chir Need 3: 25–37, 1951.
40. Ruud JT: The ice fish. Sci Am 213: 108–114, 1965.
41. Buckberg GD, Dyson CW, Emerson RC: Techniques for administering clinical cardioplegia – blood cardioplegia. In: A Textbook of Clinical Cardioplegia, Engelman RM, Levitsky S (ed). Futura Publishing, Mt. Kisco, New York, 1982: 305–316.
42. Austen WG: Experimental studies on the effects of acidosis and alkalosis on myocardial function after aortic occlusion. J Surg Res 5: 191–194, 1965.
43. Caress DL, Kissack AS, Slovin AJ, et al.: The effect of respiratory and metabolic acidosis on myocardial contractility. J Thorac Cardiovasc Surg 56: 571–577, 1968.
44. Chesnais JM, Coraboeuf E, Sauvant MP, et al.: Sensitivity to H^+, Li^+, and Mg^+ ions of the slow inward sodium current in frog atrial fibres. J Mol Cell Cardiol 7: 627–642, 1975.
45. Clowes HA, Sanga GA, Konitoxis A, et al.: Affect of acidosis on cardiovascular function in surgical patients. Ann Surg 154: 524–533, 1961.
46. Cobbe SM, Poole-Wilson PA: The time of onset and severity of acidosis in myocardial ischemia. J Mo Cell Cardiol 12: 745–760, 1980.
47. Fry Ch, Poole-Wilson PA: Effects of acid-base changes on excitation-contraction coupling in guinea pig and rabbit cardiac ventricular muscle. J Physiol (Lond) 313: 141–160, 1981.
48. Larkovic H: Influence of changes in pH on the mechanical activity of cardiac muscle. Circ Res 19: 711–717, 1966.

49. Nahas GG, Cavert HM: Cardiac depressant effect of CO_2 and its reversal. Am J Physiol 190: 483–491, 1957.
50. Poole-Wilson PA, Langer GA: Effect of pH on ionic exchange and function in rat and rabbit myocardium. Am J Physiol 229: 570–581, 1975.
51. Poole-Wilson PA: Acidosis and contractility of heart muscle. In: Metabolic Acidosis, Ciba Foundation Symposium 87; Pitman Books, London, 1982: 58–76.
52. Subramanian S, Vlad P, Fischer L, et al.: Sequellae of profound hypothermia and circulatory arrest in the corrective treatment of congenital heart disease in infants and small children. In: The Child with Congenital Heart Disease after Surgery, Kidd BSL, Rowe RD (eds). Futura Publishing, Mt. Kisco, New York, 1976: 421.
53. Tyers FGO, Todd GJ, Niebauer IM, et al.: The mechanism of myocardial damage following potassium citrate (Melrose) cardioplegia. Surgery 78: 45–53, 1975.
54. Whelan DA Jr, Hamilton DG, Ganote E, et al.: Effect of transient period of ischemia on myocardial cells. 1. Effects on cell volume regulation. Am J Path 74: 381–392, 1974.
55. Williamson JR, Schaffer SW, Ford C, et al.: Contribution of tissue acidosis to ischemic injury in the perfused rat heart. Circulation (Supplement I) 53: 3–14, 1976.
56. Schmidt CF: The influence of cerebral blood-flow on respiration. 1. The respiratory responses to changes in cerebral blood-flow. Am J Physiol 84: 202–207, 1928.
57. Gibbs FA, Maxwell H, Gibbs EL: Volume flow of blood through human brain. AMA Arch Neuro Physchiat 57: 132–139, 1947.
58. Kety SS, Schmidt CF: The nitrous-oxide method for quantitative determination of cerebral blood flow in man: theory, procedure, and normal values. J Clin Invest 27: 475–485, 1948.
59. Parkins WM, Jensen JM, Vars HM: Brain cooling in the prevention of brain damage during periods of circulatory occlusion in dogs. Ann Surg 140: 248–255, 1954.
60. Bjork VO, Hultquist G: Contraindication to profound hypothermia in open-heart surgery. J Thorac Cardiovasc Surg 44: 1–13, 1962.
61. Brierly JB: Neuropathological findings in patients dying after heart surgery. Thorax 18: 291–299, 1963.
62. Egerton N, Egerton WS, Kay JH: Neurologic changes following profound hypothermia. Ann Surg 157: 366–374, 1963.
63. Payne WS, Theye RA, Kirklin JW: Effect of carbon dioxide on rate of brain cooling during induction of hypothermia by direct blood cooling. J Surg Res 3: 54–61, 1963.
64. Belsey RH, Dowlatshaki K, Skinner DB: Profound hypothermia in cardiac surgery. J Thorac Cardiovasc Surg 56: 497–506, 1968.
65. Swan H: Clinical hypothermia: A lady with a past and some promise for the future. Surgery 73: 736–758, 1973.
66. Ream AK, Reitz BA, Silverberg G: Temperature correction of P_{CO_2} and pH in estimating acid-base status. Anesthesiology 56: 51–44, 1982.
67. Perna AM, Gardner TJ, Tabaddor K, et al.: Cerebral metabolism and blood flow after circulatory arrest during deep hypothermia. Ann Surg 178: 95–100, 1973.
68. Hagerdal M, Harp J, Siesjo BK: Influence of changes in arterial P_{CO_2} on cerebral blood flow and cerebral energy state during hypothermia in the rat. Acta Anesth Scand Suppl 57: 25–31, 1975.
69. Carlson C, Hagerdal M, Siesjo BK: The effect of hypothermia upon oxygen consumption and upon organic phosphates, glycolytic metabolites, citric acid cycle intermediates and associated amino acids in rat cerebral cortex. J Neurochem 26: 1001–1012, 1976.
70. Barrett-Boyes BG: Discussion of Brunberg, Reilly and Doty. Circulation, Supplement II, 49 and 50: 67–68, 1974.
71. Brunberg JA, Reilly E, Doty DB: Central nervous system consequences in infants after cardiac surgery using deep hypothermia and circulatory arrest. Circulation, Supplement II, 49 and 50: 60–68, 1974.
72. Clarkson PM, MacArthur BA, Barrett-Boyes BG, et al.: Developmental progress after cardiac

106

72. Clarkson PM, MacArthur BA, Barrett-Boyes BG, et al.: Developmental progress after cardiac surgery in infancy using hypothermia and circulatory arrest. Circulation 62: 855–961, 1980.
73. Lincoln C, Wells F, Coghill S, et al.: Intelligence quotient and development following use of profound hypothermia and circulatory arrest for the repair of congenital heart defect in infants and young children. J Thorac Cardiovasc Surg. In press.
74. Wolfson SK Jr, Valow EH, Eisenstat S: Temperature differentials and metabolism in profound hypothermia. JAMA 183: 674–679, 1963.
75. Brettschneider H Jr, Hubner G, Knoll D: Myocardial resistance and tolerance to ischemia: Physiological and biochemical basis. J Cardiovasc Surg 16: 241–260, 1975.
76. Buckberg GD, Brazier JR, Nelson RL, et al.: Studies of the efects of hypothermia on regional blood flow and metabolism during cardiopulmonary bypass. J Thorac Cardiovasc Surg 73: 87–95, 1977.
77. Gay WA Jr, Ebert PA: Functional, metabolic and morphological effects of potassium-induced cardioplegia. Surgery 74: 284–290, 1973.
78. Hearse DJ, Steward DA, Brainbridge MV: Myocardial protection during ischemic cardiac arrest. Importance of magnesium in cardoplegic infusates. J Thorac Cardiovasc Surg 75: 875–877, 1978.
79. Jynge P, Hearse DJ, Brainbridge MV, et al.: Myocardial protection during ischemic cardiac arrest. J Thorac Cardiovasc Surg 73: 848–855, 1977.
80. Kirsch V, Rodewald G, Karlmar P: Induced ischemic arrest. J Thorac Cardiovasc Surg 63: 121–128, 1969.
81. Bhayana JN, Gage AA: Intraoperative myocardial protection by potassium arrest and local cardiac hypothermia. Cryobiology 16: 526–533, 1979.
82. Ellis R, Ebert PA: Advantage of hypothermia and potassium cardioplegia in left ventricular hypertrophy. Ann Thorac Surg 24: 299–306, 1977.
83. Follette DM, Mulder DG, Maloney JV Jr, et al.: Advantages of blood cardioplegia over continuous coronary perfusion or intermittent ischemia. J Thorac Cardiovasc Surg 76: 604–619, 1978.
84. Roe BD, Hutchinson JC, Fishman NH, et al.: Myocardial protection with cold, ischemic potassium-induced cardioplegia. J Thorac Cardiovasc Surg 73: 366–376, 1977.
85. Cox JL, Sabiston DC Jr: Electro-physiologic consequences of cardioplegic preservation, ischemia, and reperfusion. In: A Textbook of Clinical Cardioplegia, Engelman RM, Levitsky S (eds). Futura Publishing Co., Mt. Kisco, N.Y., 1982: 405–417.
86. Clark RE, Ferguson TB, West PN, et al.: Pharmacologic preservation of the ischemic heart. Ann Thorac Surg 24: 307–314, 1977.
87. Brettschneider H Jr: Cardioplegic Workshop, Litwak RS (ed). Mt. Sinai School of Medicine, New York, 1979.
88. Blesse N, Doring V, Kalmar P, et al.: Intraoperative myocardial protection by cardioplegia in hypothermia. J Thorac Cardiovasc Surg 75: 405–413, 1978.
89. Rahn H: Body temperature and acid-base regulation. Pneumonologie 151: 87–94, 1974.
90. Litwak RD (ed): Cardioplegic Workshop. Mt. Sinai School of Medicine, New York, 1979.
91. Cross FS, Jones RD, Berne RM: Localized cardiac hypothermia as an adjunct to elective cardiac arrest. Surg Forum 8: 355–359, 1975.
92. Maloney JV, Nelson RL: Myocardial preservation during cardiopulmonary bypass. J Thorac Cardiovasc Surg 70: 1040–1049, 1975.
93. Cunningham JN, Cantinella FP, Spencer FC: Blood cardioplegia – experience with prolonged cross-clamping. In: A Textbook of Clinical Cardioplegia, Engelman RM, Levitsky S (eds). Futura Publishing Co., Mt. Kisco, N.Y., 1982: 241–264.
94. Buckberg GD: Reply to the editor. J Thorac Cardiovasc Surg 85: 148–149, 1983.
95. Swain JA: Letter to the editor. J Thorac Cardiovasc Surg 85: 147–148, 1983.
96. Swan H: The hydroxyl – hydrogen ion concentration ratio during hypothermia. Surg Gynecol Obstet 155: 897–912, 1983.
97. Kindig NB, Filley GF: Graphic representation of CO_2 equilibria in biologic systems. Physiol Teacher 26: 304–309, 1983.

6. Hypothermia and acid-base regulation in infants

O. PRAKASH, B. JONSON and S.H. MEIJ

Introduction

Hypothermia has a long history in medicine, and has been used as a remedy for diseases on the basis of its known effects and also on purely hypothetical assumptions. In ancient times, Hippocrates described the use of ice for controlling hemorrhage, a treatment that is still in frequent use. 'Refrigeration' was used by Baron Lary, Napoleon's surgeon, to carry out surgical interventions on soldiers. Local cooling by evaporating ether for local anaesthesia was already in use in the middle of the last century, a principle still employed in the form of ethyl chloride spray. Total body cooling was first applied on the basis of ideas that are today regarded as non-rational, e.g., by James Currie in 1798 [1] for febrile disease, and by Talbott [2] as a form of shock therapy in psychotic patients.

Modern use of total body hypothermia is based on an increasing knowledge of the physiological reactions to hypothermia that has been accumulating since the time when Walther in 1862 [3] and Claude Bernard in 1876 [4] made their studies in this field. The rationale for the use of total body hypothermia in modern anaesthesia is to reduce metabolism so that circulation can be reduced, or even stopped, for the period of time needed to perform the intended surgery. The use of whole body hypothermia was first developed in the 1950's in neuro- and cardiac surgery. This presentation will focus on cardiac surgery, and particularly on hypothermia applied to such a degree that circulation can be completely stopped for an hour, or even more, in infants.

As early as in 1949, McQuiston [5] advocated total body cooling during surgery of children with cyanotic heart disease. Bigelow showed in 1950 [6] that dogs cooled by immersion in cold water tolerated circulatory arrest for 15 minutes. Lewis and Tauffic [7] stopped circulation at 28°C for 15 minutes in infants undergoing repair for atrial septal defects in 1952. Later on, the development of cardiopulmonary bypass and selective cardiac hypothermia and cardioplegia added new aspects, such as the possibility of rapid cooling and re-warming, and improved preservation of the myocardium. Improved perfusion techniques did not, however, lead to abandonment of profound hypothermia with circulatory arrest. This technique is increasingly applied for the repair of congenital defects in infants [8–12].

We know very little about the rate of metabolism and about the intracellular events in an infant without circulation or any other vital sign at a temperature of about 15° C. The passage from 37° C to the lower temperatures and back to 37° C is engendered by complex physiological events. The following text will analyze some features of this complex pattern to explain alternative clinical strategies to be followed when an infant is passing through the temperature zones. Problems exist, both as to modes to produce hypothermia and to monitor and maintain a status that preserves functional integrity until the infant is safely returned to a temperature of 37° C.

Physiological reactions to hypothermia

Aerobic metabolism

The prime goal of hypothermia is to depress aerobic metabolism. Shivering is an important factor working against this goal, and it must be controlled by pharmacological paralysis during cooling and re-warming. Anaesthesia must also be given in a form that does not give unnecessary sympathetic stress that also will tend to maintain a high metabolic rate. Smith and Fay [13], who applied hypothermia as a treatment of malignant disease in 1940, were the first to realize the need for muscle relaxants and anaesthesia. Anaesthesia probably depresses the hypothalamic control of the body temperature.

In a study in which proper consideration to these factors was given, it was shown that O_2-consumption. $\dot{V}_{O_2}$, and CO_2-production, $\dot{V}_{CO_2}$, fell at a similar rate during so-called 'body surface cooling' [12]. RQ remained constant, which indicated that body stores of CO_2 were reasonably constant, a factor that will be discussed below. $\dot{V}_{O_2}$ showed small fluctuations, with a cycle time of about 1 minute, and large fluctuations about every 5 minutes. $\dot{V}_{CO_2}$ fluctuated synchronously, but to a lesser degree. This pattern was consistently observed. The reasons for these cyclic variations in aerobic metabolism reflecting O_2-uptake are not known. The damping of the CO_2-fluctuation is explained by the larger CO_2-stores in blood and tissues acting as a buffer between the sites of production and the lungs.

The CO_2-production was estimated according to the equation: $\dot{V}_{CO_2}/Wt = 0.416 \times T - 7.573$ where Wt is body weight in kilograms; T is core temperature; $\dot{V}_{CO_2}$ is in ml $CO_2 \cdot kg^{-1} \cdot min^{-1}$. The coefficient of variation was about 15% at all temperatures beteen 22° and 37° C. At a core temperature of 25° C measured in the oesophagus, aerobic metabolism is about one-third of that at 37° C.

Data from later studies (vide infra) showed that surface cooling produces considerable temperature gradients in the body. The periphery is colder than that measured in the core. In a given compartment or tissue, the relation between aerobic metabolism and temperature is probably not linear. These new considerations contradict our previous suggestion that the metabolism should take new pathways at very low temperatures [12]. No data are available on the rate and nature of metabolism at a temperature around 16° C, prevailing during circulatory arrest in man, though Benazon in 1960 [14] showed that metabolism continues at a very slow rate.

Circulation

An intense peripheral vasoconstriction is caused in part by central sympathetic activity, and in part by local reaction to cold. By increasing insulation, vasoconstriction will retard the process of surface cooling. Low peripheral circulation promotes large temperature gradients between periphery and core, the latter zone lagging behind. During cooling, renal blood flow falls, as does renal oxygen consumption and tubular function. The kidneys response to ADH stimulation is reduced [15]. Sodium reabsorption is completely inhibited at 28–18° C [16]. This factor and glucosuria may lead to polyuria.

During surface cooling, the cardiac output and heart rate fall, if anaesthesia holds back stress reactions. The heart function is extremely dependent upon acid base status, as has been discussed elsewhere in this book. In our experience, based upon the acid-base strategy of 'constant relative alkalinity', we do not generally observe gross widening of QRS-complexes, pronounced ST-T changes, ventricular arrhythmia or so-called Osborn waves [17]. Supraventricular arrhythmia is common, particularly below 25° C, but circulation is otherwise stable. The release of lactate during cooling and re-warming in our studies is small, signifying that circulation is adequate to prevent anaerobic metabolism. In this context, it is worthwhile to point out that the leftward shift of the oxygen dissociation curve of haemoglobin at low temperatures has not been shown to lead to tissue hypoxia, as has sometimes been postulated [18].

Cellular loss of potassium during deep hypothermia has under some circumstances been shown to produce cardiac rhythm disturbances [19–21]. In our series, plasma potassium, sodium, calcium and chloride concentrations did not change appreciably when they were studied during surface cooling at temperatures down to about 25° C. Blood glucose levels rise during hypothermia. The stress of induced hypothermia in the absence of efficient anaesthesia can cause glucogenolysis and gluconeogenesis from stimulation of adrenal catecholamines and glucocorticoids. Hypothermia produces reduced insulin activity [22–24]. There is a general reduction in liver function and a reduction of glycogen stores. A depletion of easily available body stores of fat, carbohydrate and protein follows progressive hypothermia and is related to the release of cortisol, catecholamines and other stress hormones.

Clinical concepts for induced hypothermia

Acid-base status

In most blood gas laboratories, blood is analyzed at 37° C. Rosenthal showed in 1948 [25] that if blood is taken from a patient with a lower temperature, the pH will fall 0.015 units per degree Centigrade when the blood is warmed to 37° C. Confusion exists over how to report data and how to interpret the status when the patient's temperature differs from 37° C. Three various ways exist according to Becker [26]:

1. A correction factor for pH is applied, and efforts are made to keep the pH at 7.4, at the patient's temperature.
2. No correction factor is used; the goal is to maintain pH at 7.4, as it is measured at 37° C and reported uncorrected.
3. pH is kept even higher than corresponding to 7.4, as measured at 37° C.

The first approach means that $PaCO_2$ has to be maintained at about 40 mm Hg at low temperatures, despite the low $\dot{V}_{CO_2}$. This is usually achieved by adding CO_2 to the ventilator or heart-lung machine. Considering that the neutrality point shifts towards higher pH-values at lower temperatures, the strategy of constant pH is equivalent to a 'relative acidosis'. The shift of the neutrality point is 0.017 units per degree Centigrade (see Chapter 2).

The second approach, at which the measured uncorrected pH is maintained at 7.4, means that the real pH of the patient goes up by 0.015 per degree Centigrade, so as to maintain a 'constant relative alkalinity' for extracellular fluids (see Chapter 1).

The third principle, called 'the concept of relative alkalosis', means that the pH of the patient is allowed to increase still more at falling temperatures than 0.017 per degree Centigrade. This principle was introduced by Mohri *et al.* [27] and is described in Chapter 6.

Since the procedure of profound hypothermia for cardiac surgery in infants was started in Rotterdam, adherence to the strategy of constant relative alkalinity has been the goal. The reasons are:

1. Normal pH at 37° C is about 7.4 in blood and about 0.6 units lower in the cells. The cell interior is close to a pH of 6.8, which is the point of electrochemical neutrality at 37° C [28]. To maintain constant relationships to neutrality, the pH at 25° C should be about 7.6 in the blood and 7.0 in the cells.

2. When blood under physiological conditions is cooled on its way from core to, e.g., a cold hand, pH changes occur that are in accordance with a constant relative alkalinity. This effect of the strong buffering action of the imidazole group of histidine means that a pH of 7.4 is not the only physiological pH in man or any other animal. Lessons learned from our cold-blooded ancestors speak in support of this [29].

3. The protein net charge and the function of most enzymes are maintained in an optimal way.

4. Donnan's equilibrium over cell membranes will not be disturbed.[1]

5. CO_2-stores are stable. If the strategy of 'constant relative alkalinity' is successfully followed, CO_2-stores will be unchanged. This means that expired CO_2 represents CO_2 production that can thus easily be measured to illustrate the metabolic depression. A strategy of constant pH implies that CO_2-stores increase at low temperatures and that large amounts of CO_2 must be eliminated during rewarming. Re-warming via a heart-lung machine is very fast (Fig. 1). The difficulties in maintaining a desired P_{CO_2} and pH are then great if a constant pH is desired.

6. It is an easy strategy to follow. Several factors make the strategy of constant alkalinity easy. The fall in metabolism and CO_2-production with temperature means that the constant ventilation established at 37° C will cause a fall of alveolar and arterial P_{CO_2}. This reduction and the associated changes in pK and CO_2 solubility increase blood pH and maintain a constant relative alkalinity and alpha-stat [28, 30] without change in plasma bicarbonate of CO_2 stores [31, 32]. The principle of normothermic ventilation is hence to adjust the ventilator at 37° C and keep it at that level while the temperature falls during cooling, and to resume the same ventilation during the warm-up period.

7. Experimental and clinical evidence support the strategy. Initial results based upon a normothermic ventilation during cooling and re-warming and a pH-regimen that followed the concept of constant relative alkalinity [12] have been confirmed by postive clinical experience in about 400 cases. Recent studies of the stability of heart rhythm [35], cardiac function, and perfusion of vital organs such as the brain [26] provide evidence that a constant pH strategy, i.e. relative acidosis at low temperatures, is deleterious. The latter study [26] also shows that a relative alkalosis is still better than constant relative alkalinity in puppies.

An important factor to realize is that this principle is a basis that cannot be adhered to blindly. Physiological dead space may increase during cooling and put extra demands on ventilation, although such changes are as a rule small [12]. The rate at which $\dot{V}_{CO_2}$ falls in relation to core temperature shows individual variations. Hence, we follow the principle of normothermic ventilation supported by Rahn and co-workers [28, 33], but finally set the ventilation according to continuous measurements of core temperature and expired CO_2, and intermittent measurements of arterial pH and P_{CO_2} during cooling and re-warming of infants.

Blood is analyzed at 37° C. The data for pH, P_{CO_2} and BE are not corrected to the body temperature when they are used for maintenance of proper acid base status. The data are regarded as if they were taken at 37° C. For physiological calculations, proper conversions to the body temperature are, of course, applied [25]. When the blood is warmed in the analyzer, the P_{CO_2} will increase because of the lower solubility of CO_2, and pH will fall. An example: Blood taken at 25° C, at which temperature P_{CO_2} is 24 mm Hg and pH is 7.6, will after re-warming give a

---

1. Points 1–4 are fully discussed in other chapters of this book.

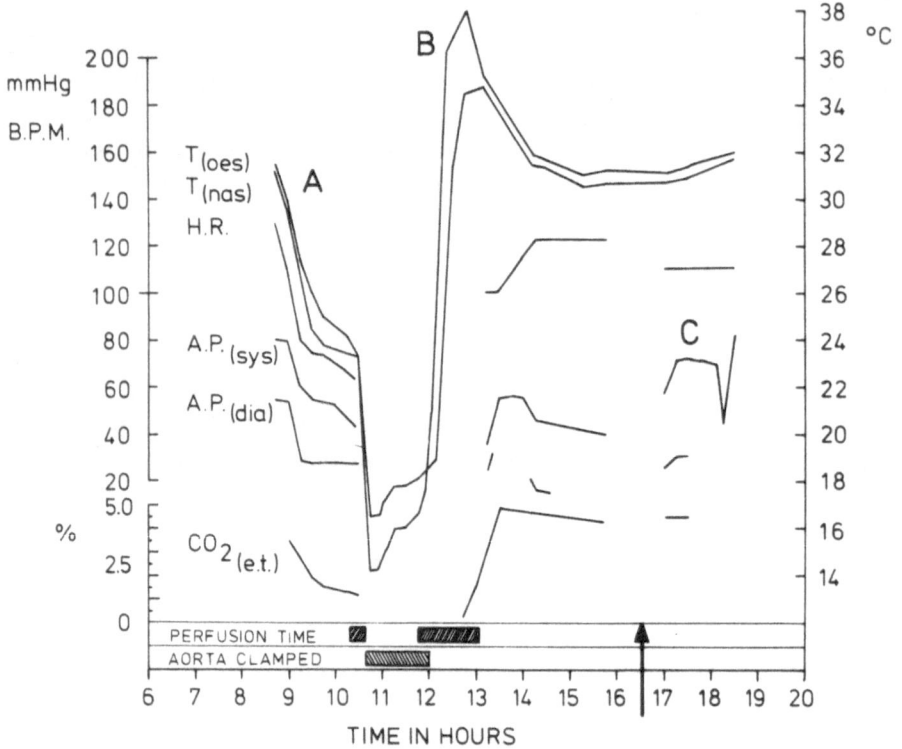

Fig. 1. Typical chart A) during cooling, B) during re-warming and C) in the post-operative period. Oesophageal temperature, T(oes), nasopharyngeal temperature, T(nas), heart rate, HR, systolic arterial pressure, A.P. (sys), diastolic arterial pressure A.P.(dia) and end-tidal CO_2-concentration are displayed. Note that CO_2-elimination via the lungs starts as soon as the heart starts beating. At the arrow, the patient was transferred to the postoperative unit.

P_{CO_2} of 40 mm Hg and a pH of 7.4. The P_{CO_2} of 24 and the pH of 7.6 are regarded as ideal at 25° C. This is easy to see from the normal blood gas data as they appear at 37° C.

In a recent review, Ream *et al.* [34] did not identify 'any investigator who is willing to offer a rebuttal, based upon experimental data, to abandoning correction for acid base management'.

Techniques of cooling

There are two principal strategies for cooling applied in pediatric anaesthesia for cardiac surgery. One is based on initial surface cooling and final cooling by cardiopulmonary bypass. The second is based upon core cooling by cardiopulmonary bypass alone.

Body surface cooling can be accomplished by immersion in pure cold water or by packing the infant in ice. It has the theoretical advantage of cooling the peripheral tissues first, so that their metabolism and circulation are efficiently depressed before heart function and central circulation decline. Also, a source for undesired reheating of the core is abolished, as long as the periphery is cooler than the core. Surface cooling alone has not, in man, been brought down to temperatures around 16° C that are needed for circulatory arrest.

Early studies indicated very high risks of ventricular fibrillation at temperatures below 28° C, and heart standstill at temperatures lower than that. Even if such risks are greatly reduced when the concept of constant relative alkalinity is applied, we do not know the risks of surface cooling to temperatures below 25–20° C.

A phenomenon that warrants caution exists in infants with the tetralogy of Fallot, and other vitia with similar haemodynamics. A pronounced right-to-left shunt may develop at core temperatures between 25 and 29° C. At transpositions with a high initial right-to-left shunt, the reverse phenomenon is observed, i.e. the shunt tends to fall during cooling.

Surface cooling is a slow, inefficient process, particularly as circulation through peripheral tissues is decreased. For these reasons, surface cooling is followed by final core cooling before circulatory arrest is begun.

Core cooling via a heart-lung machine is, with modern techniques, a quick and efficient method to produce hypothermia. The speed has in many centres become an important argument for core cooling when facilities for surgery must be efficiently utilized to meet increasing demands. It gives optimal protection against heart arrhythmia and other circulatory risks during cooling. A major drawback is its longer perfusion periods and an increased risk for haematological complications.

In order to elucidate the advantages with either method of cooling, Eberhart *et al.* [36] studied a sub-human primate, the macaque monkey. The temperature was continuously measured prior to, during and following a hypothermic arrest period at 16 positions. The cooling was done with core cooling alone, and with surface-core cooling.

All sites at which temperature was measured intracranially followed the same course during core cooling, circulatory arrest and re-warming. The temperature of the tympanic membrane is representative for intracranial temperatures.

The temperature gradients within the body as a whole after core cooling were large. Many tissues underwent the arrest period at relatively high temperatures. In the high temperature zones, metabolism may be depressed to a suboptimal degree, and may produce potentially harmful metabolites, accumulating in the tissues. This may increase the risk for cellular damage. Wash-out of metabolites after cooling from such warmer regions may, during the re-warming phase, increase the risk for malfunction of other organs.

During the period of circulatory arrest of slightly more than 30 minutes, the intracranial temperatures rose by about 5° C because of conductance from other organs and from the surroundings.

When surface cooling was followed by core cooling, the total cooling process took a longer time. The perfusion time was shorter. The temperature gradients within the body were smaller after final cooling. During the period of circulatory arrest, cranial temperatures did not rise – rather, they fell slightly.

In conclusion, studies by Eberhart *et al.* [36] confirm the advantages of surface cooling that previously were postulated. The physiological advantages of surface cooling, however, have not been proven to yield better clinical results. The practical advantages of primary core cooling may therefore warrant the use of this method. It would appear that further clinical studies are needed to settle the issue about the optimal method of cooling. One aspect of the problem that we find very important to stress is: If surface cooling is applied, the concept of constant relative alkalinity must be applied to ensure optimal function of vital organs during the procedure, and the safety of the patient (vide infra).

Techniques applied for profound hypothermia and surface cooling at our Centre

Anaesthesia techniques

No premedication is given. Anaesthesia is induced by cyclopropane in oxygen and continued by i.v. injection of fentanyl ($5 \mu g/kg$) and pancuronium ($0.2 mg/kg$). 50% nitrous oxide, 40% oxygen and 10% nitrogen are given. Nitrogen is added to reduce tendencies towards overexpansion or collapse of poorly ventilated lung units during nitrous oxide wash-in or wash-out.

The ventilation, adjusted at the initial core temperature of $35-36°C$, is not systematically changed during cooling or re-warming, nor is CO_2 added to the respiratory circuit. To prevent lung collapse, $2-3 cm H_2O$ of positive end expiratory pressure (PEEP) is applied after opening the chest.

Surface cooling is performed by placing the child on a cooling blanket and covering the entire body surface with bags of crushed ice. Heparin, $3 mg/kg$, is given before the patient is further cooled on cardiopulmonary bypass. No CO_2 is added to the pump.

Extracorporeal circulation for core cooling and re-warming

The extracorporeal circulation is maintained by a Sarns roller pump, a Temptrol Q 130 oxygenator and a Pall millipore blood filter in the arterial line. The circuit is primed with 1000 ml of a mixture of Haemaccel (Behring Pharma) and fresh heparinized blood. The amount of Haemaccel is adjusted to provide a perfusion hematocrit of about 30%. K^+ is added to give $2-3 mEq/l$ and HCO_3^- is added to give $20-40 mEq/l$ to the perfusate, depending on preperfusion levels. The core cooling is continued until the temperature is below $16°C$.

The average period of total circulatory arrest is about 50 minutes and can range from 20 to 110 minutes. After intracardiac repair, cardiopulmonary bypass is reinstituted. Perfusion for re-warming is continued until oesophageal and naso-pharyngeal temperatures reach 36° C. The average time for re-warming is about 50 minutes (range 30–75 minutes).

The re-warming should proceed cautiously. The temperature gradient between warm blood in heart-lung machine and patient should not exceed 10° C. The warming blanket bath should be warmed to 37° C. In most of the patients, defibrillation occurs spontaneously when heart temperature is about 28° C. Re-warming is quicker with pulsatile flow. It has been observed that the patients cool off after discontinuation of bypass at 36° C, when cool peripheral tissues begin to equilibrate with the warm perfused core. Further re-warming should proceed by surface means and the patient's own mechanism of maintaining temperature. Heparin reversal by slow injection of protamine should proceed cautiously. Fresh frozen plasma or fresh blood for transfusion helps in the coagulation process.

Ventilation and monitoring system

Blood gases and pH in arterial blood (PaO_2, $PaCO_2$ and pHa) are intermittently measured at 37° C, as the body temperature is lowered (ABL 2, Radiometer). Oxygen saturation in arterial blood (SaO_2) is determined intermittently with hemoreflector (American Optical Co., Massachusetts). Temperature is continuously measured in the nasopharynx, oesophagus and rectum.

A Servo Ventilator 900C, containing transducers for airway flow and pressure [37], is connected to the lung mechanics unit 940 [38] and the CO_2-analyzer 930 [12]. (All of these units from Siemens-Elema). The lung mechanics unit gives data on compliance and resistance of the respiratory system. The CO_2-analyzer displays six derived variables, such as end tidal CO_2 percentage and carbon dioxide minute production in ml/min ($\dot{V}CO_2$). For detailed measurements of both O_2-consumption and CO_2-production, a mass spectrometer can be used (Perkin Elmer, MG 1100 A). Airway flow and pressure, expired CO_2, mass spectrometer signals, arterial and central venous pressure and ECG are continuously recorded on a multichannel recorder (Hewlett-Packard).

Monitoring and control of ventilation

The standards of ventilation that maintain carbon dioxide and oxygen home-ostatis have been studied by several investigators. Radford [40, 41] presented ventilation standards which are based on predictions of CO_2-production and dead space from a patient's sex, body weight and predictable changes in basal meta-

116

bolic rate caused by elevation in body temperature. The accuracy of his ventilation standards has been confirmed by others [42, 43]. When these standards are applied to infants below 10 kg and under 1 year of age they are not useful. It is rather embarrassing to see that ventilation during anaesthesia and critical care is too often controlled by manual methods and by the intuition of physicians, nurses and respiratory technicians or from some normothermic estimations of metabolism.

In infants undergoing a hypothermic procedure, special means for proper control of ventilation are necessary for several reasons. Arterial P_{CO_2} must be accurately and continuously estimated to ensure optimal heart function. The size of the infant (from about 3 to 10 kg) means that a large fraction of tidal volume is lost due to gas compression in the ventilator and the series dead space.

Measurements of expired CO_2 have long been found useful to adjust ventilation to demands [44, 45, 46]. Arterial P_{CO_2} corresponds closely to end tidal P_{CO_2} in the absence of large degrees of ventilation/perfusion abnormalities. Measurements of end tidal P_{CO_2} then allow a proper means to adjust ventilation so that the desired PaCO$_2$ is maintained.

When, however, high frequency and a low tidal volume are used, or when ventilation/perfusion inequalities are pronounced [46, 47, 48], end tidal gas may not be representative for average alveolar and arterial P_{CO_2}. West [49] used a digital computer to calculate the dead space ratio (V_D/V_T) that would result from uneven ventilation/perfusion. He showed that there was a strong positive correlation between the two phenomena.

The single breath analysis for CO_2 in which expired CO_2-fraction is plotted against expired volume is a means for a more detailed exploration of the information available. The single breath tracing (Fig. 2) can be divided into three phases [50]. Phase I is the CO_2-free phase or absolute dead space [51], representing gas

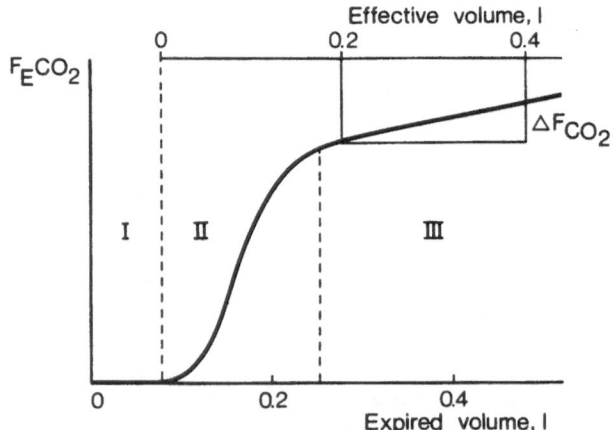

Fig. 2. The three phases of the single breath test. Phases II and III can be called the effective volume [46]. The slope of the alveolar plateau, ΔF_{CO_2}, is an index of uneven ventilation/perfusion [48].

from the airways. Phase II is characterized by a rapid S-shaped upswing in the tracing, representing (a) the wash-out of the convective airway with alveolar gas, and (b) the 'progressive recruitment of transit times' [52]. Phase III represents alveolar gas, and has been called the alveolar plateau; it usually ascends gradually.

The single breath test for CO_2 has been used in our studies since 1974 [12]. Its use in anaesthesia has been explored on the basis of detailed theoretical analysis in a thesis by Fletcher [48]. In the present context, a description of a system for monitoring ventilation based on CO_2-analysis is warranted.

Monitoring equipment designed to measure expired CO_2 in infants

The CO_2-unit has a sensor and a calculator. The former (Fig. 3) is an infrared CO_2-meter, comprising a cuvette and a photometer. The cuvette is a chamber with two windows. The cuvette is connected to the Y-piece for connection of the patient to the ventilator. The cuvette is placed in the light-path so that one window in its wall faces an infrared emittor and the other window an infrared sensor. The cuvette can be removed from the photometer for cleaning. The light from an infrared emitter is chopped at the frequency of 180 Hz. On the opposite side of the cuvette, there is a photodiode conducter which senses the light at a wave-length of 4.2 μm. At this wave-length, no gas in common use will directly

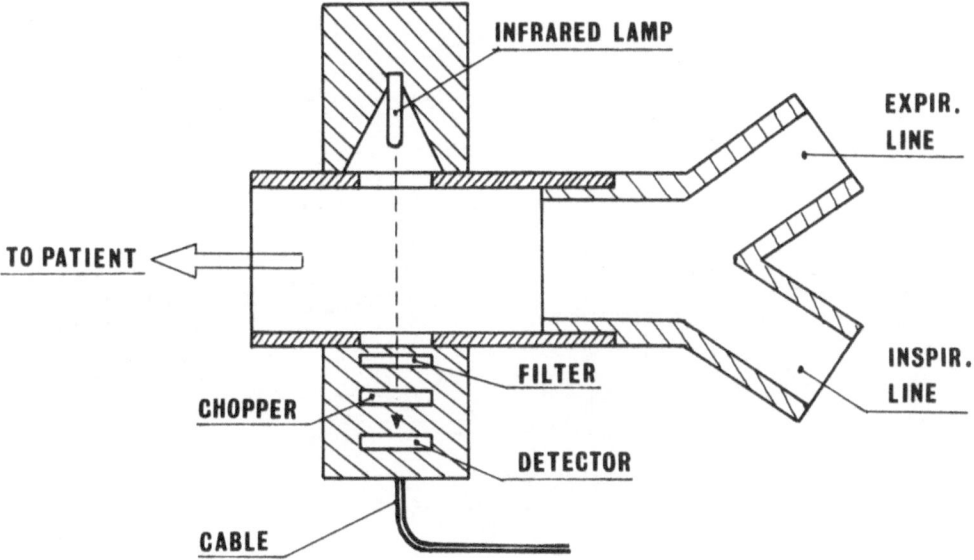

Fig. 3. The 'cuvette' constitutes a Y-piece connecting the expiratory and inspiratory lines with the patient. The cuvette is placed in the light path so that one window in its wall faces a pulsed infrared emittor and the opposite window an infrared sensor.

affect the signal significantly. Collision broadening, however, caused by N_2O, will affect the calibration of the CO_2-unit. Calibration at the existing barometric pressure with gas with known fraction of CO_2 and with N_2O-O_2 in the proportion used during anaesthesia will solve these problems. The simultaneous flow signal is obtained from the Servo Ventilator. The ventilator calibration is checked against a wet gas meter. Wet gas meters have been shown to be acceptably accurate in the presence of N_2O [53]. CO_2 is, thus, sensed in the main stream of gas as closely as possible to the patient. The principle infers that the change of CO_2-concentration will be recognized extremely fast. The 100% response time is about 20 ms.

No condensation will occur within the sample cuvette while it is heated. The sensor is $2 \times 3 \times 7$ cm, and weighs 190 g. The sampling cuvette has a dead space of 5 ml, and if attached to connectors suitable for infants-tubing, the dead space is 4 ml. The dead space is smaller than the ordinary Y-piece that it replaces. The resistance of the sampling cuvette is 0.8 cmH$_2$O/(l/s) at a flow rate of 0.5 l/s, and is thus negligible.

The calculator is attached to the Servo Ventilator and to the sensor (Fig. 4). From the former, it obtains a signal representing expiratory flow rate, $\dot{V}_E$, inspiratory flow rate, $\dot{V}_I$, power, and timing pulses telling when expiration starts and ends, and from the latter a signal corresponding to CO_2-fraction, F_{CO_2}.

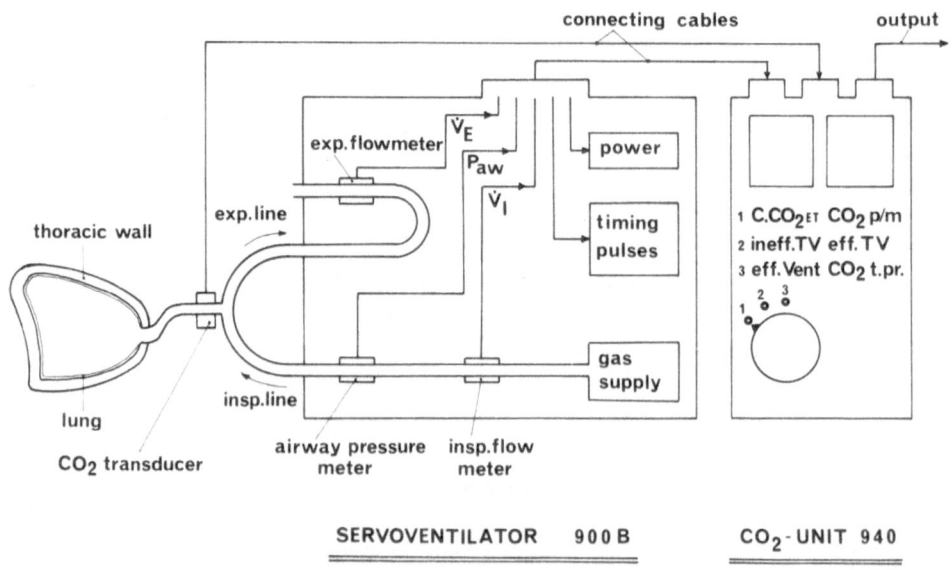

Fig. 4. Schematic view over lungs and airways, with the CO_2-sensor, the CO_2-unit and the ventilator.

Principle of calculations

The instantaneous flow of CO_2 is calculated as the product between volume flow rate, $\dot{V}_E$ and F_{CO_2}:

$$\dot{V}_{CO_2} = \dot{V}_E \times F_{CO_2}$$

Some problems will occur as $\dot{V}_E$ is not measured at the patient, but within the ventilator. As the air in the inspiratory and expiratory lines is compressible, an error will occur. The error is small and can be observed only at the start of inspiration when there is some CO_2-rich gas in the Y-piece, and when there is a rapidly rising pressure in the lines. The small negative flow of CO_2 observed at the start of inspiration (Fig. 5) is thus to some extent an artefact. Because of the dead space (5 ml), some CO_2 will, however, return to the patient.

As the dead space of the cuvette is very small, the error will have little importance. It could be further reduced by not calculating influx of CO_2 to the patient, as is the case with new CO_2-analyzers from Siemens-Elema. The feature of our older equipment where influx is counted is valuable if a leakage of the inspiratory should occur. This line will then be filled by expired gas reinsufflated during the following inspiration, which will immediately show up in the tracing of $\dot{V}_{CO_2}$.

Volumes of CO_2 transferred from (and to) a patient are calculated by integration of $\dot{V}_{CO_2}$ (Fig. 5). $\dot{V}_{CO_2}$ is read by a memory at the end of the expiration to provide a continuous signal corresponding to $\dot{V}_{CO_2}$ eliminated during the last breath, i.e., tidal CO_2-volume, $\dot{V}_T CO_2$. The $\dot{V}_T CO_2$ signal is fed to an averaging circuit that supplies a signal of the volume of CO_2 eliminated per minute.

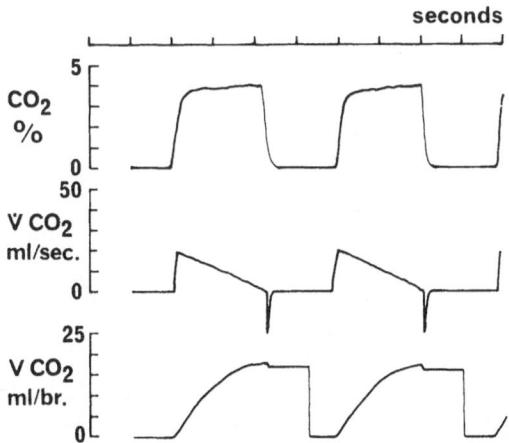

Fig. 5. Tracings from the CO_2-unit.

120

The single breath tracing

Initially, an oscilloscope was used to display F_{CO_2} against expired volume [12]. We have later developed a device which consists of a microprocessor and a display unit. The microprocessor system converts the analog signals ($\dot{V}_E$, F_{CO_2}) from the ventilator to digital data and feeds this digital information to a display unit, such that a continuous display of the single breath test for CO_2 is presented on the screen. The microprocessor system also has the capability of freezing a particular pattern for making photographs such as that shown in Fig. 6.

As was previously shown, the niveau of the alveolar plateau fell with temperature along with the lower CO_2-production. No important change in the shape occurred. No change is seen with respect to airway dead space, and only little change is observed when physiological dead space is calculated from $PaCO_2$ [12]. As mentioned earlier in this paper, all signals from the ventilator and CO_2-unit and/or mass spectrometer are recorded on an analog tape recorder. Thus, we are able to reproduce the single breath tracings off line on our larger computer systems. An example of the latter is shown in Fig. 7. It shows the tracings of an infant at 5 months of age, with a VSD at the end of the surface cooling period (T = 24° C) and after the operation at the end of re-warming (T = 35.5° C).

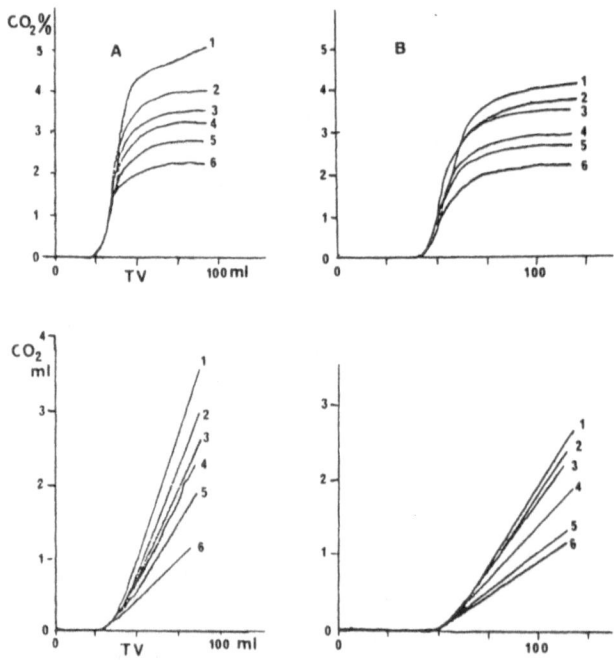

Fig. 6A – B. Examples of on-line single breath traces during surface cooling from different patients: top, CO_2 % against tidal volume, bottom, CO_2-production against tidal volume (TV). A. Panels show tracings from an infant of 8.5 kg with Fallot's tetralogy. Tracings 1–6 represent the cooling process from 35° C to 25° C. B. Tracings from an infant with transpositions of the great vessels during cooling.

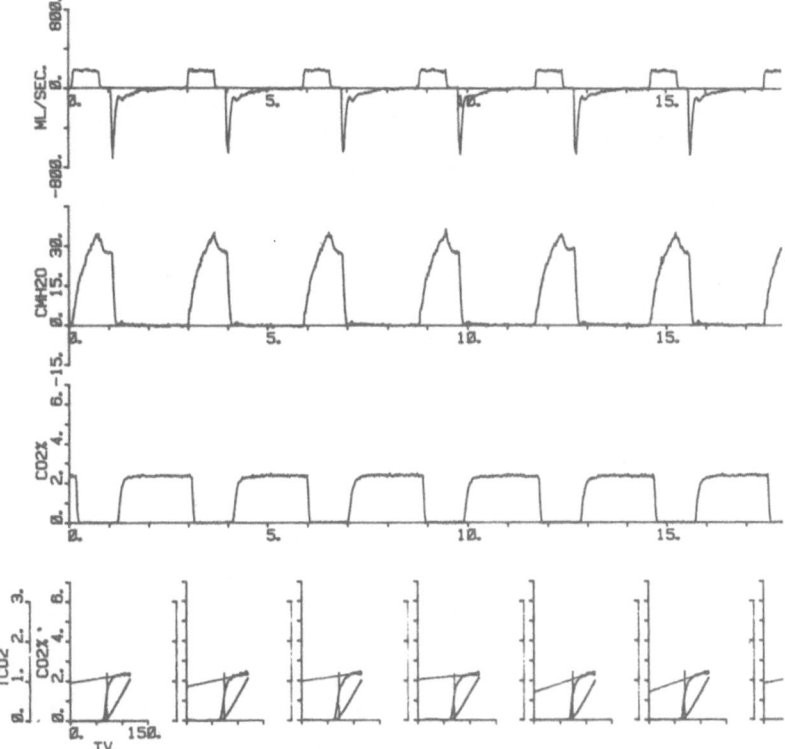

Fig. 7A. Example of off-line traces during surface cooling. From top to bottom: airway flow, airway pressure, CO_2-concentration against time and at bottom, single breath curves of CO_2 % and tidal CO_2-production, TCO_2 in ml, plotted against tidal volume, TV.

Usefulness of CO_2-monitoring

Continuous monitoring of gas exchange has several purposes. It provides protection against ventilatory or circulatory catastrophes; it also allows adjustment of ventilation and it offers a tool for studies of clinical procedures.

Protection against catastrophes

Any event leading to sudden disturbance of the ventilation or perfusion of the lungs can be detected by gas-exchange studies. Disconnections or blockage of ventilatory tubings, severe airways obstruction, pneumothorax, bleeding, the surgeon's manipulations with the heart and the great vessels and heart arrhythmias are common problems. Examples have been published previously [54]. Early detection of raised metabolism gives early warning of hyperpyrexia.

Increased security is gained only if the signal is available immediately and all

122

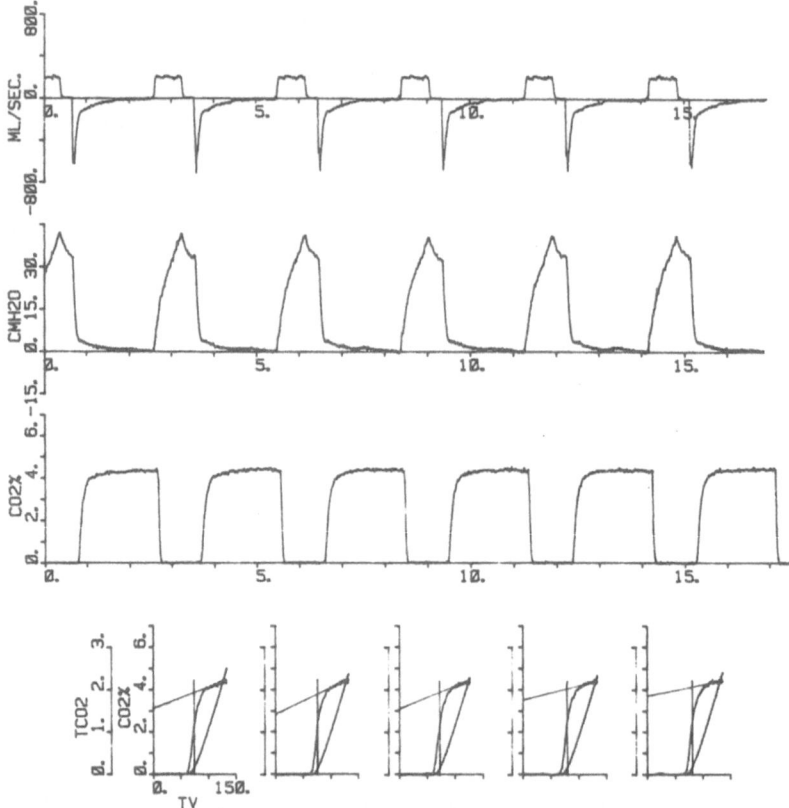

Fig. 7B. Same as in 7A, but after re-warming.

the time. This means that the equipment may not take up too much space, or be too cumbersome to use, and cannot be shared by several users. The immediate sensing of CO_2 in the infant makes it possible to analyze $\dot{V}_{CO_2}$ breath-by-breath and improves speed compared to systems based on mixing of expired gas. The CO_2-unit that not only measures CO_2 but also integrates this measurement with the flow-signal from the ventilator represents a step forward in our efforts to provide for compact and easy-to-use equipment. The microcomputer system enhances the usefulness of CO_2-monitoring considerably, as it provides graphic information from which deviating patterns are easily detected.

Adjustment of ventilation during cooling

Immediately at the start of anaesthesia, ventilation can be adjusted on the basis of end-tidal CO_2. During surface cooling, the end-tidal CO_2 and $\dot{V}_{CO_2}$ fall in accordance with the concept of constant relative alkalinity. Table 1 illustrates how arterial and expired CO_2-values should change during cooling according to this

Table 1. Average arterial and end-tidal CO_2-values in infants cooled by surface cooling according to the concepts of constant relative alkalinity. The table starts at 35°C, as infants usually spontaneously drop to that temperature during preoperative preparations. The data are based on references 12 and 29.

Body temperature, °C	35	30	25
$PaCO_2$ mm Hg (corrected to body temp.)	35	26	18
End-tidal CO_2 % (barometric pressure 750 mm Hg)	4.0	2.8	1.7
$\dot{V}_{CO_2}$, % of initial value	100	70	40

concept. As discussed earlier, most infants follow this course without changes of their ventilation, but deviations occur. When this is observed, signs of disturbed circulation should be searched for, and an arterial sample taken. The treatment is then corrected on the basis of all observations made. Adjustment of ventilation may be needed. Core cooling by perfusion may be indicated if signs of disturbed circulation, e.g., right-to-left shunting, are seen.

When end-tidal CO_2 approaches 2.5 or 2% according to the particular case, or when core temperature reaches 25°C, the chest is opened and cannulation for extracorporeal circulation performed. Sometimes the core temperature reaches 20°C before core cooling without any adverse effects.

Re-warming

During re-warming via perfusion, the heart usually starts to contract regularly without defibrillation [12]. A proper acid-base strategy is certainly a prerequisite for this [26, 35, 55, 56]. Ventilation is resumed when re-warming starts. As soon as heart action starts, CO_2-elimination should be seen to increase. The relationship between left and right atrial pressures representing preload of the ventricles, and CO_2-production representing cardiac output gives an immediate impression of heart function. One can even, by rapid changes of blood volume in the patient via the heart-lung machine, change preload and immediately see the response of heart-action in terms of $\dot{V}_{CO_2}$. This form of Starling test of the heart is only possible with equipment that gives $\dot{V}_{CO_2}$ on a breath-by-breath basis. Should $\dot{V}_{CO_2}$ not reach reasonable levels towards the end of re-warming and at an adequate preload, proper continued diagnostic and therapeutic measures should immediately be carried out.

Acid base status is a key issue during this very dynamic period, when tissues are being re-perfused and may release, e.g., lactate, particularly when circulatory arrest has been very long. This is, however, no great problem in our unit, as intervening periods of perfusion seem to be most effective when longer ptriods of circulatory arrest are required for cardiac repair. Immediae access to blood gas data is very important, as is continuous CO_2-monitoring.

Postoperative period

Infants, in particular, often need prolonged postoperative artificial ventilation. We ventilate them on an average for 35 hours. This period is characterized by large variations in aerobic metabolism due to reversal of anaesthesia and sedation and to continuing changes in temperature and activities. During the period of artificial ventilation, a continuous monitoring, including expired CO_2, is for us of central importance. Figure 8 illustrates the course in an infant operated for VSD at seven months of age. On arrival at the ICU, the rectal and particularly the peripheral skin temperatures were low. This is at least partially due to incomplete re-warming by perfusion of peripheral tissues. Even core temperature fell during the first period after perfusion, a phenomenon analogous to the 'after drop' that is observed after accidental cooling [57].

During the following hours temperatures rose, CO_2-elimination increased by about 50% and ventilation had to be adjusted to the increasing demands. Just before midnight (24 h), ventilation was changed and end-tidal CO_2 fell as intended. The fall of end-tidal CO_2 should, however, be accompanied by a transient increase of $\dot{V}_{CO_2}$ resulting from wash-out of CO_2 from blood and tissues. This expected change was not observed. Rather, $\dot{V}_{CO_2}$ as well as peripheral skin temperatures fell. These undesired changes indicate that circulation was depressed by the increased ventilation. Reduced peripheral metabolism and CO_2-accumulation are responsible for the fall of $\dot{V}_{CO_2}$. A stepwise reduction of ventilation restored the situation.

Towards the end of the period of artificial ventilation, spontaneous ventilation was tested, during which $\dot{V}_{CO_2}$ increased due to the work of breathing. Because end-tidal CO_2 did not rise to unacceptable levels, extubation was performed.

The example illustrates that end-tidal CO_2 is useful for adjusting ventilation to changing demands, but requires corrections in complicated cases. Thus, measurements of $\dot{V}_{CO_2}$ are very important, as are temperature measurements and other indices of circulation.

Follow-up studies

An efficient monitoring system used in the daily routine and systematic storage and retrieval of data on a computer system are essential for a continuing follow-up of clinical activities. Recently, we analyzed the data restrospectively in a group of 25 infants undergoing total correction of congenital heart defects. The diagnosis included; 9 ventricular septal defects, 13 transpositions of the great vessels and 3 tetralogies of Fallot (weight ranged from 3130 to 7500 g and age from 1 to 17 months). All of these patients survived cooling, surgery and postoperative care. Most of them were seen regularly over a period of eight years. Their performance in schools and behaviour at home were normal, as their parents recounted it.

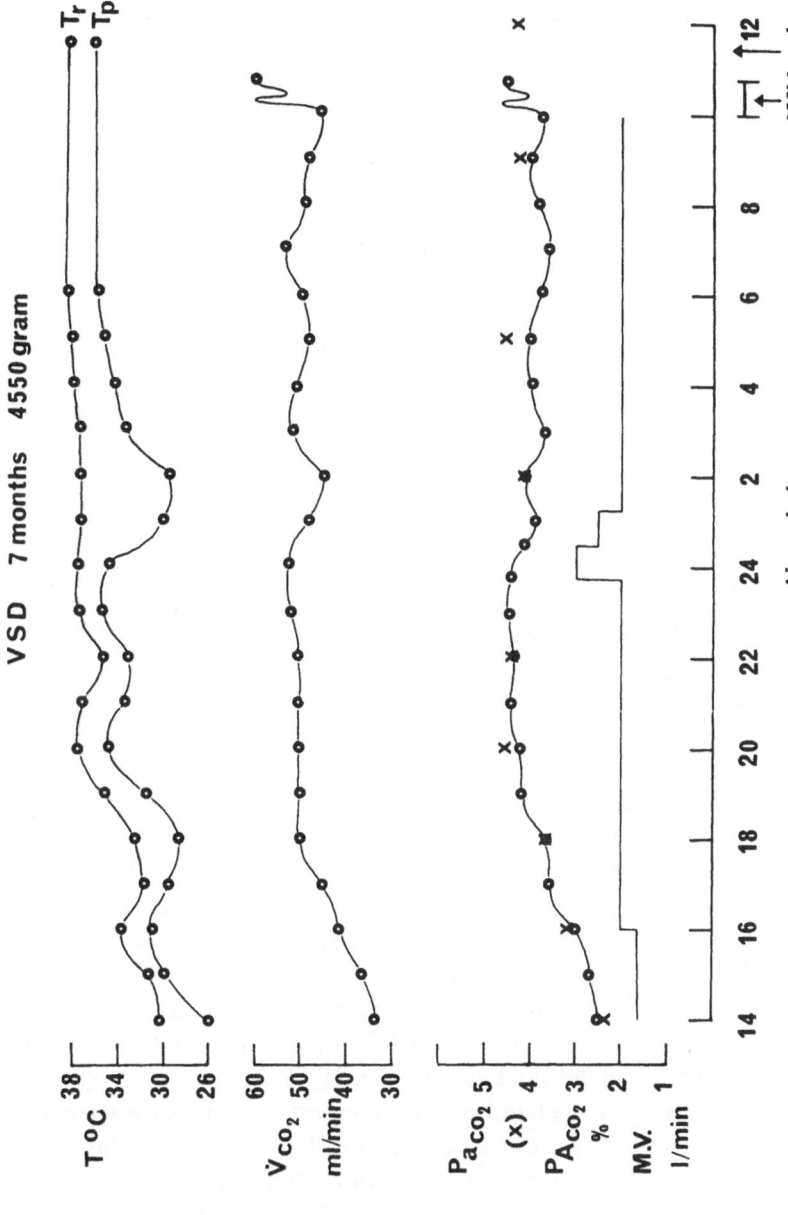

Fig. 8. Diagram showing 24 h tracings of temperature (rectal and peripheral), CO_2-elimination, arterial and alveolar P_{CO_2} and minute volume. Details are explained in the text.

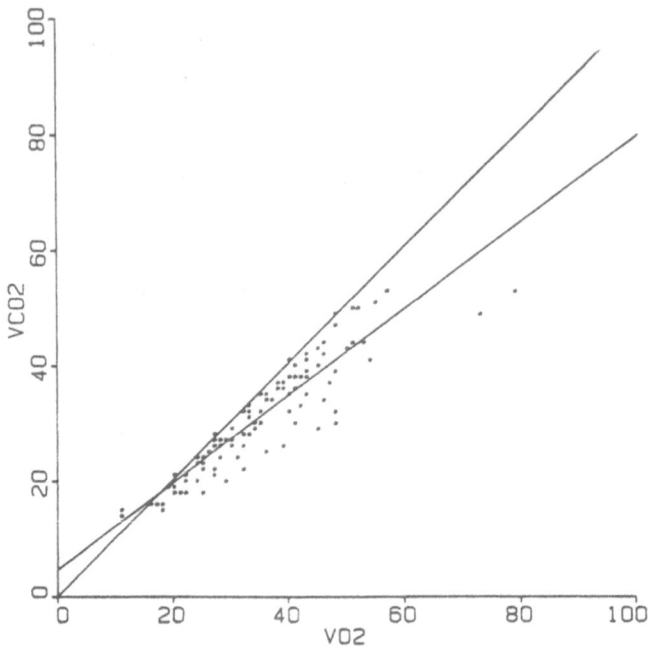

Fig. 9. O$_2$-uptake ($\dot{V}O_2$) and CO$_2$-elimination ($\dot{V}_{CO_2}$) were closely related. Line of identity, corresponding to a respiratory quotient of 1.0, and the regression line are drawn.

$\dot{V}_{O_2}$ and $\dot{V}_{CO_2}$ were strongly correlated to one another before and during surface cooling (Fig. 9). During surface cooling, $\dot{V}_{CO_2}$ fell in proportion to $\dot{V}_{O_2}$; the coefficient of correlation calculated for each infant averaged 0.97 (S.D. = 0.04). The temperature dependence of the $\dot{V}_{CO_2}$ per kg body weight (wt) in the total material can be described by $\dot{V}_{CO_2}/wt = 0.37 \times T - 5.58$ (Fig. 10). After chest closure at a core temperature of 35–36°C, the $\dot{V}_{CO_2}$ returned to 8.0 ml · min^{-1} · kg^{-1}, as compared to 8.1 before cooling. Temperature-corrected values for PaCO$_2$ fell during cooling according to: PaCO$_2$ = 1.39 T − 12.54. The coefficient of correlations for single infants was on the average 0.95 (S.D. = 0.08).

In general, temperature-corrected PaCO$_2$-values were about 4 mm Hg higher than the corresponding end-tidal values (Fig. 11). When uncorrected values for PaCO$_2$ and pHa were correlated against temperature, no significant changes were observed (Table 2). Lactate levels did not change during cooling (1.1 ± 0.4 mmol/l), but during re-warming the concentration reached a peak of 3.2 ± 0.2 mmol/l. During cooling, heart rate fell linearly (Fig. 12).

During cooling, there was no significant change in airway peak pressure or of resistance and compliance of the respiratory system. After re-warming, however, peak pressures rose from 27 before cooling to 33 cm H$_2$O (p<0.001). There was a significant increase in pHa from 7.36 to 7.47 (p<0.01) when comparing values after rewarming against the values in the evening of the same day, while the other

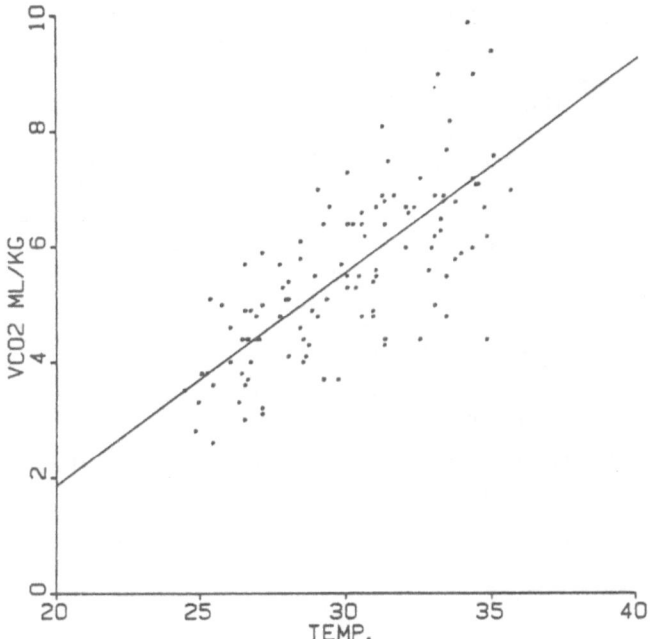

Fig. 10. CO_2-elimination in ml · min^{-1} · body w^{-1} plotted against the core temperature during surface cooling. The regression line is: $\dot{V}_{CO_2}/wt = 0.37 \times T - 5.58$.

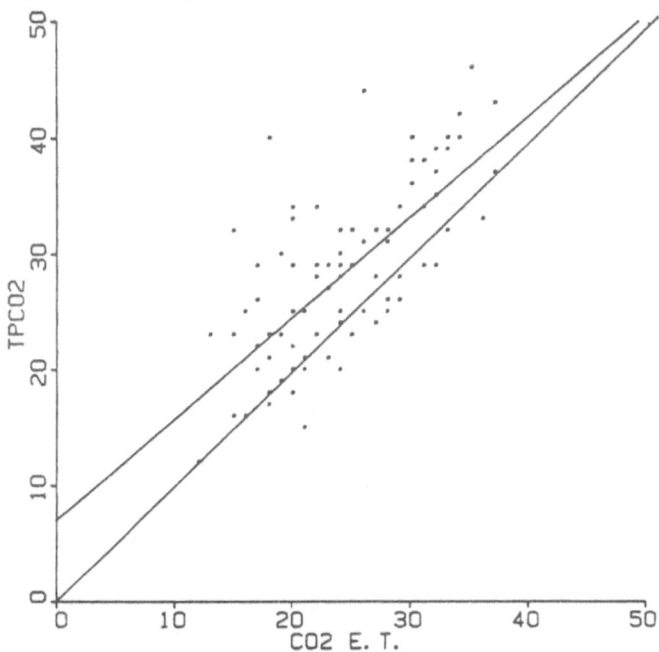

Fig. 11. Temperature-corrected $PaCO_2$-data, $TPCO_2$, plotted against the corresponding end-tidal P_{CO_2}, CO_2 E.T. $TPCO_2$ was about 4 mm Hg higher than end-tidal P_{CO_2}. Line of identity and the regression line: $TPCO_2 = 7.01 + 0.87 \times P_{CO_2}$ e.t. are drawn.

128

Table 2. Data from the cooling period and immediately after re-warming. Mean values ± SEM are given. Blood gas data are not corrected to body temperatures.

Temp °C	34°C	30°C	26°C	35°C
SaO$_2$ %	90 ± 3	85 ± 3	81 ± 4	90 ± 2
PaO$_2$ mm Hg	108 ± 21	100 ± 13	105 ± 16	84 ± 8
PaCO$_2$ mm Hg	40 ± 2	40 ± 2	37 ± 2	40 ± 2
pHa	7.36 ± 0.03	7.35 ± 0.03	7.36 ± 0.03	7.35 ± 0.01
B.E. mmol/l	−3.4 ± 1.2	−3.7 ± 1.1	−4.6 ± 1.0	−3.2 ± 0.5
Lactate mmol/l	1.1 ± 0.1	1.1 ± 0.1	1.2 ± 0.1	3.2 ± 0.3
P$_{CO_2}$ e.t. mm Hg	31 ± 1	26 ± 1*	19 ± 1*	33 ± 1
P$_{CO_2}$ (a-et) mm Hg	3 ± 1	4 ± 1	5 ± 1	4 ± 1

* $p < 0.001$, in comparison to data at 34° C.

values were stable (Table 3). The average ventilation time in the postoperative care unit was 35 hours (range: 3 hours–3 days).

Comments

The results of the follow-up study are similar to those previously reported [12]. This means that the adherence to the strategy of constant relative alkalinity was

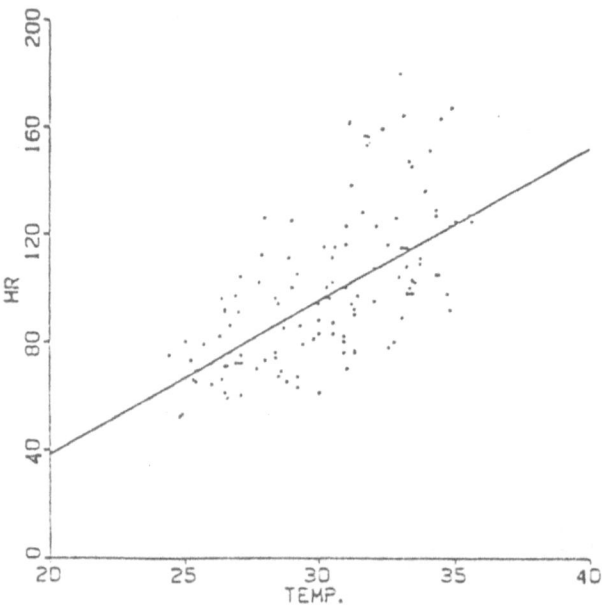

Fig. 12. Heart rate (HR) plotted against the corresponding body core temperature during surface cooling. The regression line is: HR = 5.72 × T − 76.4.

Table 3. Data from 16 infants who were ventilated until the first postoperative morning. Mean values ± SEM are given.

	Before cooling	After re-warming	Same day at 8.00 p.m.	Next morning at about 9.00 a.m.
SaO$_2$ %	90 ± 3	90 ± 2	91 ± 3	91 ± 3
PaO$_2$ mm Hg	104 ± 23	85 ± 11	81 ± 9	76 ± 9
PaCO$_2$ mm Hg	40 ± 3	40 ± 2	36 ± 2	34 ± 1
pHa	7.36 ± 0.04	7.36 ± 0.02	7.47 ± 0.02[+]	7.51 ± 0.01
BE mmol/l	−3.2 ± 1.5	−3.0 ± 0.6	2.8 ± 0.8[+]	4.5 ± 0.5
P$_{CO_2}$ e.t. mm Hg	31 ± 2	32 ± 2	33 ± 1	32 ± 1
P$_{CO_2}$ (a-et) mm Hg	3 ± 2	4 ± 0.18	5.8 ± 15	4 ± 1

[+] p<0.01 in comparison with values before cooling.

achieved according to our principle. The indices of lung function showed that lung function was at least as well preserved as in the previous study [12].

A system such as that behind surgical corrections of heart vitia in infants is a very complex one. Frequent changes in various routines, both large and small, are the result of rapidly continuing development. Some changes are initiated to improve care, others to improve efficiency. Data of the kind reported in this section permit continuous control during cooling and re-warming. It is important to emphasize that clinical routines and monitoring systems are so designed that data can be retrieved and analyzed without too much difficulty. One of the goals behind our system was to make this possible.

Concluding remarks

Profound hypothermia with total circulatory arrest was based on pioneering work done in the 1940's and 1950's [5–8, 58, 59]. In 1963, Horiuchi *et al.* [60] reported results from 78 infants radically operated for VSD under hypothermia and total circulatory arrest. The outcome was excellent, particularly in relation to poor results from surgery in infants below 10 kg in weight, with conventional cardiopulmonary bypass. Since then the method has been adopted and studied in respect to cardiovascular and other physiological effects of hypothermia in many centres [61–64].

Physiological studies in many animals and in infants undergoing surgery have been followed by an extensive discussion about the strategy of acid base balance [13, 25–35, 71, 72]. In spite of overwhelming evidence that a constant pH corrected to body temperature means physically and physiologically an acidosis leading to impaired function of vital organs during and after hypothermia, several centres have still not accepted a strategy based upon a constant relative alkalinity.

While we can hope that a reconsideration in this matter will come, the scientific

130

frontline should focus on other questions. For example, should constant relative alkalinity be adopted in other fields of medicine? Blayo *et al.* and Fox *et al.* have provided an answer in regard to adult patients undergoing hypothermia for cardiac surgery [73, 74]. They report data showing a corrected pH that rises at lower temperatures and $PaCO_2$-values that fall in close agreement with the strategy of constant relative alkalinity (Fig. 13). In our unit, the concept of constant relative alkalinity has been applied for adults cooled for cardiac surgery under perfusion since its inception in 1971.

Accidental drowning is a field in which we have found no systematic study on various pH-strategies. There is no reason to believe that the concept of constant relative alkalinity is not valid as a base for the therapy. One of us (O. P.) happens to have experience from a county hospital in Norway in the 1960's. Accidental cooling was commonly seen there. With the great limitation of facilities that existed there, and on the basis of intuition, rather than knowledge, an Engström

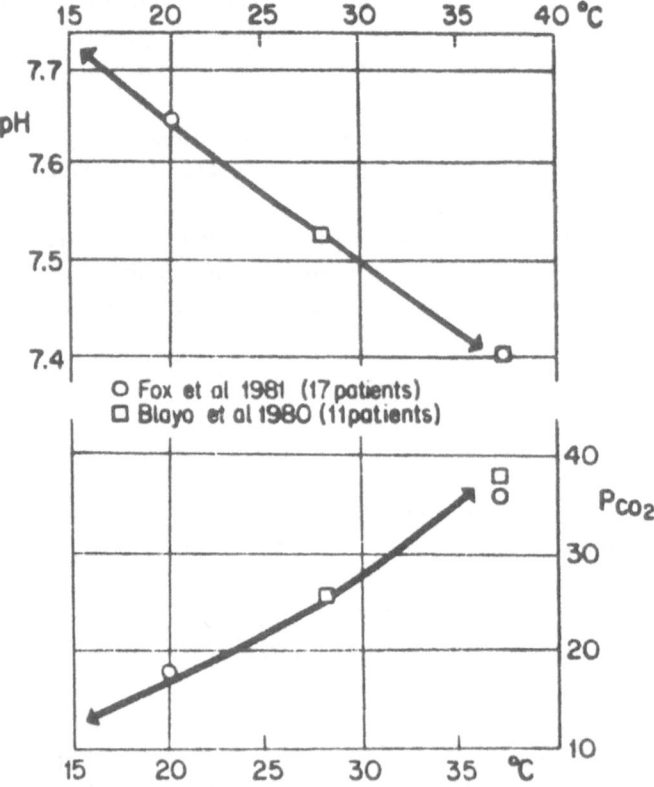

Fig. 13. Temperature-corrected arterial pH and P_{CO_2}-values reported for patients at 28° C [73] and 20° C [74]. The solid lines represent the typical behaviour of human blood when cooled anaerobically in vitro. The coincidence between the points and the solid lines indicates adherence to the concept of constant relative alkalinity. When blood of these patients is warmed, the pH and P_{CO_2}-values will follow the solid lines back to the values at 37° C, and their acid-base status can be evaluated by normal criteria. (Reproduction through the courtesy of Dr. H. Rahn.)

ventilator was used at normothermic settings. The clinical results were surprisingly good, but may be more easily understood in the light of the knowledge of today.

Another important question is: Should we go one step further and apply the concept of relative alkalosis? Systemic studies in man are needed. One may also add that a relative alkalosis may infer improved cardiac function even at a temperature of 37° C. Lachmann *et al.* studied anaesthetized dogs and found much improved cardiac function when pH was in the range of 7.5–7.6 rather than at 7.4 [75].

In critical care, we find it remarkable that in most units a pH of around 7.3 is accepted in patients with failing hearts. One hundred years after Claude Bernard, such a basic feature of the *milieu interieur* is still under poor control in our advanced care units.

References

1. Currie J. In: Medical Reports on the Effect of Water, Cold and Warm, as a Remedy in Fever and Other Disease. Codell and Davies, Liverpool, 1977.
2. Talbott JH: Physiologic and therapeutic effects of hypothermia. N Engl J Med 224: 281–288, 1941.
3. Walther A: Beiträge zur Lehre von der thierischen Wärme. Virchows Arch Path Anat 25: 414, 1862 (in German).
4. Bernard C: Le cons sur chaleur animale. Baillere, Paris, 1876 (in French).
5. McQuiston WO: Anaesthetic problems in cardiac surgery in children. Anaesthesiology 10: 590–600, 1949.
6. Bigelow WH, Lindsay WK, Greenwood WF: Hypothermia: its possible role in cardiac surgery; an investigation of factors governing survival in dogs at low body temperatures. Ann Surg 132: 849–866, 1950.
7. Lewis FJ, Tauffic M: Closure of atrial septal defects with the aid of hypothermia; experimental accomplishments and the report of one successful case. Surgery 33: 52–61, 1953.
8. Swan H, Zeavin I, Blount SG Jr, Virtue RW: Surgery by direct vision in the open heart during hypothermia. JAMA 153: 1081–1085, 1953.
9. Barratt-Boyes BG, Neutze JM, Seelye ER, Simpson M: Complete correction of cardiovascular malformations in the first year of life. Progress in Cardiovascular Diseases. Vol. XV, No. 3, Nov.–Dec., 1972.
10. Johnston AE, Radde IC, Steward DJ, Taylor J: Acid-base and electrolyte changes in infants undergoing profound hypothermia for surgical correction of congenital heart defects. Can Anaesth Soc J 21: 235, 1974.
11. Steward DJ, Sloan IA, Johnston AE: Anaesthetic management of infants undergoing profound hypothermia for surgical correction of congenital heart defects. Can Anaesth Soc J 21: 15, 1974.
12. Prakash O, Jonson B, Bos E, Meij S. et al: Cardiorespiratory and metabolic effects of profound hypothermia. Crit Care Med 6: 340–346, 1978.
13. Smith LW, Fay T: Observations on human beings with cancer: maintenance at reduced temperatures of 75–90° F. Am J Clin Pathol 10: 1–11, 1940.
14. Benazon D: The experimental and clinical use of profound hypothermia. Anaesthesia 15: 134, 1960.
15. Segar E, Riley PA, Barile TG: Urinary composition during hypothermia. Am J Physiol 185: 528, 1956.

132

16. Andjus RK, Lovelock JE, Smith AU: Resuscitation and recovery of hypothermic, supercooled and frozen mammals. Proc Nat Acad Sci (Wash.), 451: 125, 1956.
17. Osborn JJ: Experimental hypothermia: respiratory and pH changes in relation to cardiac function. Am J Physiol 175: 389, 1953.
18. Wylie WD, Churchill-Davidson HC: Hibernation and hypothermia. In: A Practice of Anaesthesia. Lloyd-Luke (Med. Books) Ltd., London, 1972: 1271–129?.
19. Fischer B, Russ C, Fedor EF, et al.: Experimental evaluation of prolonged hypothermia. Arch Surg 71: 431–448, 1955.
20. Badeer H: Ventricular fibrillation in hypothermia: Review of factors favoring fibrillation in hypothermia with and without cardiac surgery. J Thorac Surg 35: 267–273, 1958.
21. Covino BG, Hegnauer AH: Electrolytes and pH changes in relation to hypothermic ventricular fibrillation. Circ Res 3: 575–580, 1955.
22. Brown TCK, Dunlop ME, Stevens BJ, et al.: Biochemical changes during surface cooling for deep hypothermia in open-heart surgery. J Thoracic Cardiovasc Surg 65: 402–408, 1973.
23. Bickford AF, Mottran RF: Glucose metabolism during induced hypothermia. Clin Sci 19: 345–359, 1960.
24. Tyler DB: The effect of cooling on the mechanism of insulin action. Proc Soc Exp Biol Med 42: 278–280, 1939.
25. Rosenthal TB: The effects of temperature on the pH of the blood and plasma in vitro. J Biol Chem 173: 25–30, 1948.
26. Becker H, Vinten-Johansen J, Buckberg GD, Robertson JM,Leaf JD, Lazar HL, Manganaro A Jr: Myocardial damage caused by keeping pH 7.40 during systemic deep hypothermia. J Thorac Cardiovasc Surg 82: 810–820, 1981.
27. Mohri H, Dillard DH, Crawford EW, Martin WE, Merendino KA: Method of surface induced deep hypothermia for open heart surgery in infants. J Thorac Cardiovasc Surg 58: 262–270, 1969.
28. Rahn H, Reeves RB, Howell BJ: Hydrogen ion regulation, temperature and evolution. Am Rev Resp Dis 112: 165–172, 1975.
29. White FN: A comparative physiological approach to hypothermia. J Thorac Cardiovasc Surg 82: 821–831, 1981.
30. Swan H: Hydroxyl-hydrogen ion concentration ratio during hypothermia. Collective review. Surg Gynecol Obstet 155: 897–912, 1982.
31. Reeves RB: The interaction of body temperature and acid-base balance in ectothermic vertebrates. Annu Rev Physiol 39: 559–586, 1977.
32. Reeves RB, Rahn H: Patterns in vertebrate acid-base regulation. In: Evolution of Respiratory Processes: A Comparative Approach, Wood S, Lenfant C (eds). Marcel Dekker, New York, 1979: 225–252.
33. Rahn H, Reeves RB: Hydrogen ion regulation during hypothermia: from the Amazon to the operating room. In: Applied Physiology in Clinical Respiratory Care, Prakash O (ed). Martinus Nijhoff Publ., Boston, 1982: 1–15.
34. Ream AK, Reitz BA, Silverberg G: Temperature correction of P_{CO_2} and pH in estimating acid-base status; an example of the emperor's new clothes? Anesthesiology 56: 41–44, 1982.
35. Swain JA, White FN, Peters RM: The effect of pH on the hypothermia ventricular fibrillation threshold. Thorac Cardiovasc Surg 87: 445–452, 1984.
36. Eberhart RC, et al., 1982. Personal communication.
37. Ingelstedt S, Jonson B, Nordström L, Olsson SG: On automatic ventilation. Acta Anaesth Scand Suppl 47, 1972.
38. Jonson B, Nordström L, Olsson SG, Akerback D: Monitoring of ventilation and lung mechanics during automatic ventilation: A new device. Bull Phys Path Resp 11: 729, 1975.
39. Olsson SG, Fletcher R, Jonson B, Nordström L, Prakash O: Clinical studies of gas exchange during ventilatory support – a method using the Siemens-Elema CO_2 analyser. Br J Anaesth 52: 491–499, 1980.

133

40. Radford EP, Ferris BJ, Kriet BC: Clinical use of nomogram to estimate proper ventilation during artificial respiration. N Engl J Med 251: 877–884, 1954.
41. Radford EP: Ventilation standards for use in artificial respiration. J Appl Physiol 7: 451–460, 1955.
42. Etsen B, Reynolds RN, Li TH: Respiratory effects of calibrated volume limited pressure variable ventilator during surgery. J Appl Physiol 14: 736–742, 1959.
43. Nunn JF, Hill DW: Respiratory dead space and arterial end tidal P_{CO_2} tension in anesthetized man. J Appl Physiol 15: 383–389, 1970.
44. Burton GW: The value of carbon dioxide monitoring during anesthesia. Anesthesia 21: 173–183, 1966.
45. Holloman GH, Milhorn HT, Coleman TG: A sampled data regulator for maintaining a constant alveolar CO_2. J Appl Physiol 25: 463–468, 1968.
46. Fletcher R, Jonson B: Deadspace and the single breath test for carbon dioxide during anaesthesia and artificial ventilation. Br J Anaesth 56: 109–119, 1984.
47. Fletcher R, Jonson B, Cumming G, Brew J: The concept of deadspace with special reference to the single breath test for carbon dioxide. Br J Anaesth 53: 77–88, 1981.
48. Fletcher R: The single breath test for carbon dioxide. Thesis, Lund, Sweden, 1980.
49. West JB: Ventilation-perfusion inequality and overall gas exchange in computer models of the lung. Respir Physiol 7: 88–110, 1969.
50. Fowler WS: Lung function studies. V. Respiratory dead space in old age and in pulmonary emphysema. J Clin Invest 29: 1439, 1950.
51. Bartels J, Severinghaus JW, Foster RE, Briscoe WA, Bates DV: The respiratory dead space measured by single breath analysis of oxygen, carbon dioxide, nitrogen or helium. J Clin Invest 33: 41, 1954.
52. Horsfield K, Cumming G: Functional consequences of airway morphology. J Appl Physiol 24: 384, 1968.
53. Nunn JF: Respiratory measurements in the presence of nitrous oxide. Br J Anaesth 30: 254, 1958.
54. Prakash O: Monitoring of heart and lung function in cardiac surgery. Thesis, Rotterdam, 1980.
55. Turnbull AD, Dobell ARC: The effect of pH change on the ventricular fibrillation threshold. Surgery 60: 1040–1043, 1966.
56. Dong E, Stinson EB, Shumway NE: The ventricular fibrillation threshold in respiratory acidosis and alkalosis. Surgery 61: 602-607, 1967.
57. Golden FST, Herrey GR: The mechanism of the after-drop following immersion hypothermia in pigs. J Physiol 272: 26, 1977.
58. Churchill-Davidson HC, McMillan IKR, Melrose DG: Hypothermia: An experimental study of surface cooling. Lancet 2: 1011–1013, 1953.
59. Otis AB, Jude J: Effects of body temperature on pulmonary gas exchange. Am J Physiol 188: 335–359, 1957.
60. Horiuchi T, Koyamada K, Matano I, et al.: Radical operations for ventricular septal defect in infancy. J Thorac Cardiovasc Surg 46: 180–190, 1963.
61. Barratt-Boyes BG, Simpson M, Neutze JM: Intracardiac surgery in neonates and infants using deep hypothermia with surface cooling and limited cardiopulmonary bypass. Circulation 43, Suppl I, 1971 and 44: 25–30, 1971.
62. Shida H, Morimoto M, Inokawa K, Tsugane J, Ikeda Y. Simple deep hypothermia for open-heart surgery. J Cardiovasc Surg 20: 135, 1979.
63. Rudy LW, Boucher JK, Edmunds LH: The effect of deep hypothermia and circulatory arrest on the distribution of system blood flow in rhesus monkeys. J Thorac Cardiovasc Surg 64: 706, 1972.
64. Anzai T, Turner MD, Gibson WH, Neely WA: Blood flow distribution in dogs during hypothermia and post hypothermia. Am J Physiol 234: 706–710, 1978.
65. Rittenhouse EA, Ito CS, Mohri H, Merendino KA: Circulatory dynamics during surface-induced deep hypothermia and after cardiac arrest for one hour. J Thoracic Cardiovasc Surg 61: 359–369, 1971.

66. Ellis RJ, Hoover E, Gay WA, Ebert PA: Metabolic alterations with profound hypothermia. Arch Surg 109: 659, 1974.
67. McConnell DH, White FN, Nelson RL, et al.: Importance of 'alkalosis' in maintenance of ideal blood pH during hypothermia. Surg Forum 26: 263–265, 1975.
68. Howell BJ, Baumgardner FW, Bondi K, Rahn H: Acid-base balance in cold-blooded verte-brates. Proc Int Union Physiol Sc 8: 91–92, 1971.
69. Rahn H: Body temperature and acid-base regulation (review article). Pneumonologie 51: 86–94, 1974.
70. Rahn H: P_{CO_2}, pH and body temperature. In: Carbon Dioxide and Metabolic Regulation, Nahas G, Schaefer KE (eds). Springer-Verlag, Berlin, 1974: 152–162.
71. Prakash O, Jonson B, Mey S: Techniques of respiratory monitoring. Int J Clin Monit Comput 1, 1: 49–58, 1984.
72. Williams JJ, Marshall BE: A fresh look at an old question. Anesthesiology 56: 1–2, 1982.
73. Blayo MC, Lecompte Y, Pocidalo JJ: Control of acid-base status during hypothermia in man. Respir Physiol 43: 287–298, 1980.
74. Fox LS, Blackstone EH, Kirklin JW, et al.: The relationship of whole body oxygen consumption to perfusion flow rate during hypothermia cardiopulmonary bypass. J Thorac Cardiovasc Surg 83: 239–248, 1982.
75. Lachmann B, Jonson B, et al: Effects of pH 7.15 to 7.75 on cardiac output and circulatory dynamics. In: Book of Abstracts, Vol. II, the 8th World Congress of Anaesthesiologists, Manila, 1984.

7. Myocardial function resulting from varying acid-base management during and following deep surface and perfusion hypothermia and circulatory arrest

GERALD D. BUCKBERG, HEINZ BECKER,
JAKOB VINTEN-JOHANSEN, JOHN M. ROBERTSON,
JERRY LEAF, and DOUGLAS H. McCONNELL

Abstract

This study compares the systemic and cardiac effects of three different pH strategies during surface and perfusion cooling. In six adult dogs we compared the constant pH (acid) strategy to the alkaline pH strategy during perfusion hypothermia ($28°$ C). In 28 puppies we compared the constant α (neutral) pH strategy to the alkaline strategy during surface and perfusion hypothermia circulatory arrest for 1 hour, and subsequent rewarming. In 14 puppies (6 sufface and 8 perfusion) pH was kept at 7.4 (meter reading at $37°$ C) with a constant P_{CO_2} of 35–40 mmHg to follow the constant α (neutral) pH strategy. In 14 other puppies (6 surface and 8 perfusion) pH was made progressively alkalotic by reducing P_{CO_2} to 10 mmHg and adding buffer as necessary to simulate the most alkalotic range of ectotherms ($17°$ C) with a pH 7.8 meter reading at $37°$ C. All puppies underwent 1 hour of circulatory arrest with $16°$ C multidose blood cardioplegia.

In adult dogs, the alkaline strategy during perfusion hypothermia resulted in better total and regional left ventricular blood flow, higher LVO_2 uptake, better LV lactate metabolism and greater LV contratility. In puppies undergoing surface cooling, the constant α (neutral) pH strategy caused inadequate cardiac output (systemic hypotension, systemic and cardiac lactic acidosis). Conversely, the alkaline pH strategy allowed 25% higher cardiac output in normal systemic and cardiac lactate metabolism. At $22°$ C, cerebral blood flow at pH 7.4 (meter reading), P_{CO_2} 40 mmHg, fell 75% (from 26 ± 6 to 10 ± 3); however, raising pH to 7.75 (meter reading) by lowering P_{CO_2} to 10 mmHg allowed twice as much cerebral blood flow (20 ± 6 ml/100g/min). These deleterious effects of following the constant α (neutral) pH strategy were avoided during cooling and the perfusion hypothermia by ensuring organ blood flow through maintenance of adequate perfusion pressure and flow with the extracorporeal circuit. All hearts treated by the constant α (neutral) pH strategy required multiple defibrillations after circulatory and post-ischemic myocardial performance was reduced 50% and 75%, respectively, in surface and perfusion hypothermia groups. In contrast, 13 of 14 hearts defibrillated spontaneously in puppies managed by the alkaline pH strategy, and post-ischemic myocardial performance returned to normal.

We conclude that constraining pH at 7.4 (corrected or uncorrected) during hypothermia causes a degree of myocardial damage and limitation of cardioplegic protection which is avoidable by adjusting pH to a more alkaline range. These findings may have major implications in the routine management of hypothermia during all cardiac operations.

Introduction

The complexity of cardiac surgical procedures requiring surface and perfusion hypothermia makes evaluation of the role of acid-base management during cooling and rewarming difficult. In some instances, especially infants who must undergo circulatory arrest to correct complex cardiac defects, surface cooling is used to shorten the duration of cardiopulmonary bypass and provide more homogeneous organ cooling [1]. Characteristically, surface cooling is associated with reduced cardiac output, systemic lactic acidosis and ventricular fibrillation at temperatures below 28°C [2–4]. Perfusion hypothermia is used in those instances where surface cooling is not employed, or introduced usally when systemic temperature falls below 28°C with surface cooling. At 17°C, circulatory arrest is introduced and accompanied by cardioplegic myocardial protection to prevent ischemic cardiac damage. Most cardiac surgical teams keep pH and P_{CO_2} at the 'normal' values of 7.40 and 40 mmHg at all levels of hypothermia (pH constant strategy, $\Delta pH/0°C = 0.0$).

This clinical pH pattern in warm-blooded humans deviates from the pH and P_{CO_2} adjustments made by cold-blooded animals (or ectotherms described by Reeves and Rahn) who increase pH and reduce P_{CO_2} as their temperature falls [5,6] (Fig. 1). This pH pattern is termed the constant α or neutral strategy, since a constant net charge on protein is maintained over the entire temperature range when this strategy is followed. We showed previously [7] that the 28°C bypassed heart functions better if pH is adjusted to the *most* alkaline range seen in ectotherms (i.e. increasing pH from 7.37 to 7.72 or a slope of 0.033 pH units/°C, rather than at 0.017 pH units/°C slope practiced by most ectotherms (Fig. 2). This observation implies that the alkaline strategy may be applicable when euthermic animals are entered into the world of hypothermia.

This report will a) review the results of our earlier studies comparing the effects of constant pH strategy (acid) with alkaline pH strategy during perfusion hypothermia, b) summarize our recent studies comparing the alkaline pH strategy to constant α or neutral pH strategy during surface cooling followed by circulatory arrest, and c) present data during profound perfusion hypthermia and circulatory arrest where the neutral and alkaline pH strategies are compared.

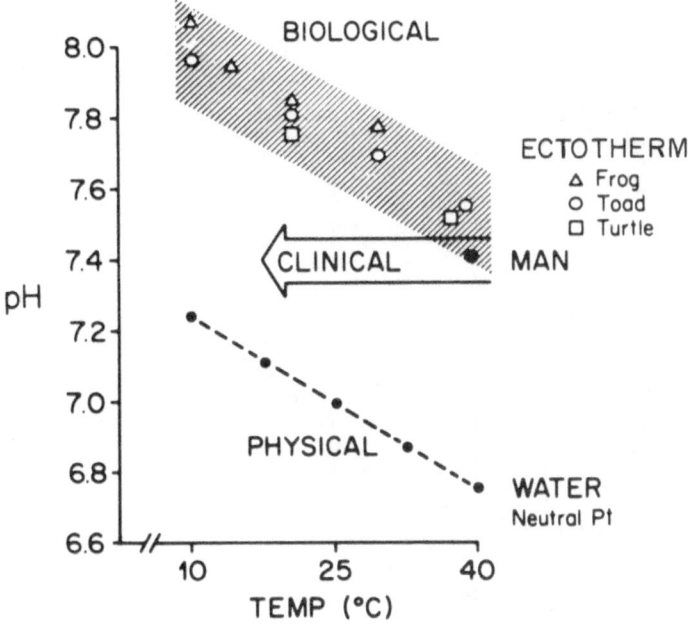

Fig. 1. Changes in pH with temperature exhibited by a) water and b) and echotherms (poikilotherms). In contrast note the pH constraint at 7.4 practiced in man in many clinical centers.

Methods

Twenty-eight puppies (6–9 kg) were premedicated with morphine sulfate (2 mg/ kg intramuscular), anesthetized with α chloralose (75 mg/kg), intubated, and breathed with room air via a Harvard respirator so that arterial pCO_2 was 35–50 mmHg. The right femoral artery and vein were cannulated for pressure monitoring and intravenous infusion. A median sternotomy was performed and the heart suspended in a pericardial cradle. Catheters were introduced into the right internal mammary artery (for microsphere collection) and into the left atrium and into the coronary sinus. The proximal aorta was dissected and a Statham electromagnetic flow meter transducer placed around the aortic root for measurement of cardiac output. Heparin (3 mg/kg) was given and cannulae placed into the left femoral artery and right atrium for subsequent induction of cardiopulmonary bypass in the event of ventricular fibrillation during immersion hypothermia. A polyvinyl catheter was placed into the ascending aorta for eventual cardioplegic administration. The azygous vein was ligated.

Immersion hypothermia was achieved by placing ice bags around the puppies and shivering was prevented with succinylcholine muscle relaxation. Perfusion hypothermia was achieved by progressively reducing blood temperature using the heater cooler in the extracorporeal circuit, while keeping the blood-core body

138

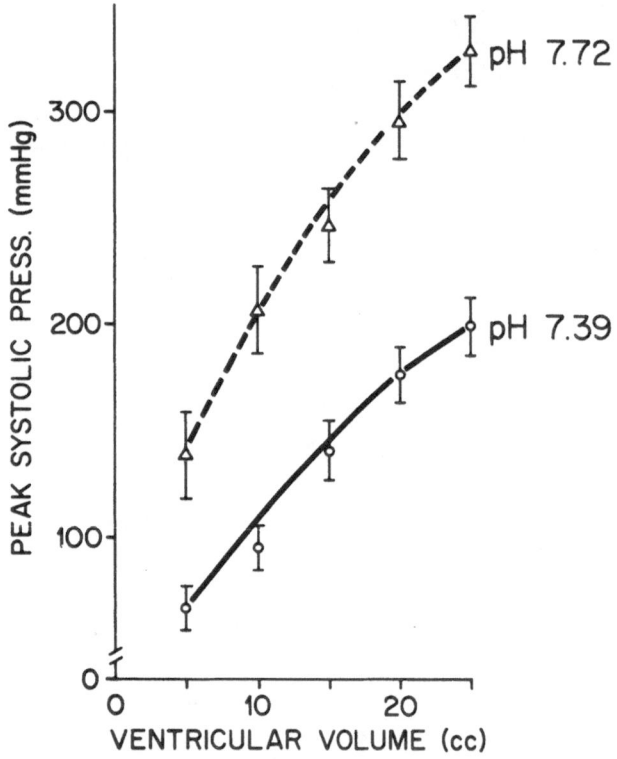

Fig. 2. Isovolumetric LV function during perfusion hypothermia (28° C) at pH 7.39 and pH 7.72 (body temperature). Note: Augmented LV performance when the alkaline pH strategy is followed in preference to the constant pH (acid) strategy.

temperature gradient at 5° C. Hematocrit was reduced from $35 \pm 2\%$ to $22 \pm 1\%$ by infusing low molecular weight dextran. Thermistor probes (Yellow Springs) were placed into the esophagus and rectum, and brain temperature was monitored with a thermistor probe placed through a small temporal cranial burr hole.

Measurements

Arterial blood was analyzed for P_{O_2}, P_{CO_2}, and pH at 37° C. pH meter reading at 37° C was recorded and then corrected for temperature by using the Rosenthal correction factor of 0.015 pH units/° C [8] (Fig. 3). Arterial, central venous and coronary sinus blood samples were analyzed for oxygen content [9] and for lactate. Total and regional blood flows were measured by injecting 15 ± 3 micron microspheres [10] labelled with either I^{125}, Ce^{141}, Sr^{85}, Sc^{46}, Sn^{115}, and Nb^{95}, while a reference sample was withdrawn simultaneously for 3 minutes. After the experiment, hearts were stopped with intracardiac injection of $MgSO_4$. The brain,

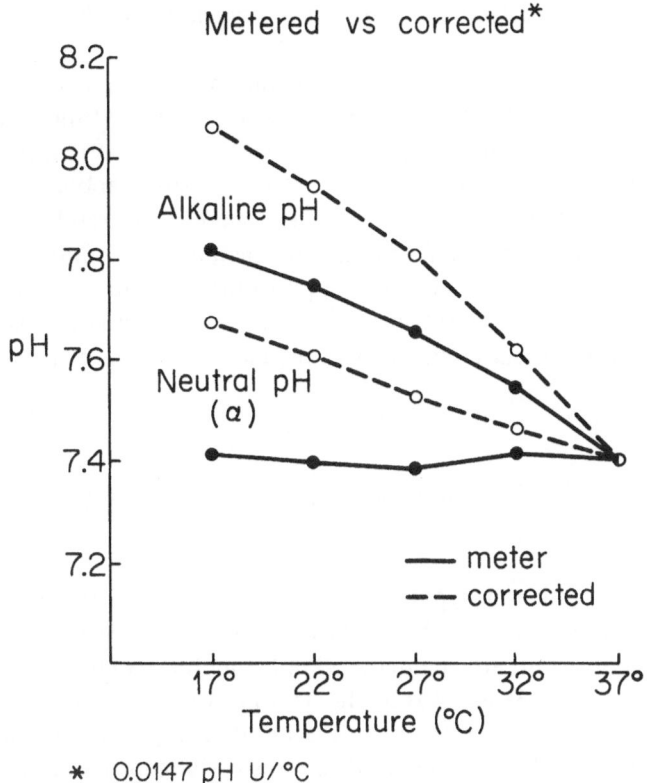

Fig. 3. Metered and corrected pH values in this study. The alkaline pH strategy refers to puppies where pH was adjusted to the upper range of values shown in Fig. 1.

heart, and kidneys were removed and divided into tared vials. Radioactive content of each nuclide was determined by gamma spectrometry, and blood flow was calculated as described previously [10]. Systemic oxygen consumption was calculated from cardiac output and arterial venous oxygen content differences. Left ventricular oxygen consumption was calculated from left ventricular blood flow and arterial-coronary sinus oxygen content differences. Similar calculations were used for lactate metabolism.

Experimental protocol

After cannulation, 20 minutes were allowed for establishment of steady state conditions at 37°C, arterial pH 7.4. Hemodynamic measurements and blood samples were obtained and the first microsphere was injected.

Constant pH (acid) vs alkaline pH strategy – perfusion hypothermia (28°)

Six adult dogs were placed on total cardiopulmonary bypass and systemic temperature lowered to 28° C. Perfusion pressure was kept at 90 mmHg and pH was varied by adjusting P_{CO_2} and adding HCO_{3-} (when necessary) from 7.39 ± 0.02 (measured at body temperature) to 7.72 ± 0.03 (measured at body temperature). Total and regional left ventricular blood flow were measured by injecting 8–10 microspheres. Left ventricular oxygen and lactate consumptions (arterial – venous × LV flow) and left ventricular performance (intraventricular balloon function curves from 0 to 25 ml volume) were measured at pH 7.40 and 7.70 body temperature. Under these circumstances the meter readings were 7.25 and 7.55, respectively, at 37° C.

Constant α(neutral) pH vs alkaline pH strategy during surface and perfusion hypothermia (to 17° C)

In 12 puppies, immersion hypothermia was begun as described and perfusion hypothermia was begun in 16 others at 80 mm perfusion pressure. In 14 puppies (6 immersion, 8 perfusion) arterial pH was kept at meter reading of 7.40 at 37° C by keeping P_{CO_2} between 35 and 40 mmHg. This group was treated, therefore, by a constant α or neutral pH strategy. In the 14 other puppies (6 immersion and 8 perfusion), arterial pH was increased progressively to produce alkalosis either through hyperventilation or by reducing P_{CO_2} in the extracorporeal circuit to a minimum of 10 mmHg to maintain pH in the very upper range of ectothermic values (Fig. 1); aliquots of $NaHCO_3$ or Tham were added when necessary. This upper range was selected because our previous study showed best myocardial performance to occur at these levels during perfusion hypothermia [7]; this strategy can be termed the alkaline pH strategy.

Cardiac output (or pump flow), arterial pressure, heart rate and rectal, esophageal, and brain temperatures were recorded continuously. Measurement of organ blood flow (microspheres), systemic and coronary sinus oxygen and lactate content were made at 37° C, 32° C, 27° C, 22° C, and following rewarming. Equivalent amounts of donor blood or dextran were given to replace blood samples. Extracorporeal circulation was started in the puppies undergoing surface cooling when rectal temperature reached 22° C or when spontaneous ventricular fibrillation occurred, and lowered further to 17° C by perfusion hypothermia. Small aliquots of Tham or $NaHCO_3$ are added if pH does not reach the desired level at the different temperatures.

At 17° C systemic temperature (brain, rectal, esophageal), the aorta was clamped and blood cardioplegic arrest instituted by delivering 350 ml of our standard blood cardioplegic solution [11] at 16° C using the delivery system reported previously [11]. Simultaneously, total circulatory arrest was achieved by stopping the

arterial pump of the extracorporeal circuit and allowing the puppies to exsangui-
nate into the oxygenator. Each 20 minutes of circulatory arrest, 250 ml of 16° C
blood cardioplegic replenishment was given into the proximal aorta.

After 56 minutes of circulatory arrest, the blood in the extracorporeal circuit
was recirculated and warmed to 24° C. At 60 minutes, the 24° C extracorporeal
circulation was restarted. Simultaneously, we delivered a 24° C blood cardioplegic
reperfusate into the proximal aorta at 50 ml/min over 5 minutes and removed the
aortic clamp. In 14 puppies, arterial pH was kept at 7.4 (meter reading at 37° C)
throughout rewarming to follow the constant α (neutral) pH strategy. In the 14
others, pH was lowered progressively by adding CO_2 to achieve the values during
cooling. Defibrillation, when necessary, was done when fibrillation became
vigorous. Body temperature was increased to 37° C and final measurements made
30 minutes after aortic unclamping.

Results

Results are shown in Fig. 2–13 and Tables 1–4.

Constant pH (acid strategy) vs alkaline pH strategy – perfusion hypothermia

Raising blood pH from 7.40 to 7.70 resulted in a 65% (p<0.01) increase in total
left ventricular flow and augmented subendocardial flow 50% (p<.01) (Fig. 4).
This increased flow was accompanied by an 81% rise (p<.01) in left ventricular
oxygen uptake and a 210% increase (p<.01) in myocardial lactate utilization
(Figs. 5, 6). There was no anaerobic cardiac metabolism in these studies of
perfusion hypothermia where the extracorporeal circuit kept perfusion pressure
at 90 mmHg. The increased metabolic rate and myocardial perfusion occurring

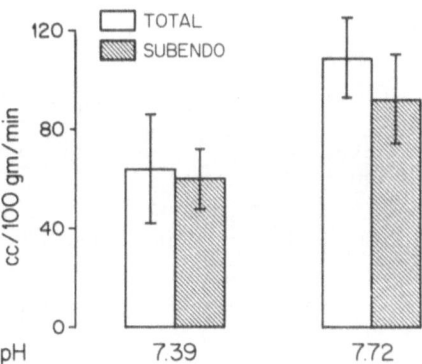

Fig. 4. Total and regional LV flow. Adult dogs during perfusion hypothermia (28° C) where the
constant pH (7.39) and alkaline (7.72) pH strategies are compared. See text for description.

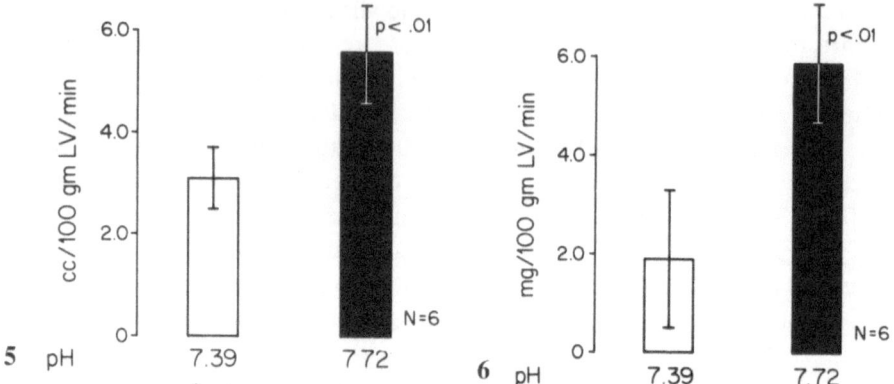

Fig. 5. Left ventricular oxygen consumption per minute during perfusion hypothermia (28°C) in adult dogs where the constant pH (acid) strategy and alkaline strategies are compared.

Fig. 6. Left ventricular lactate consumption per minute in adult dogs during perfusion hypothermia (28°C) where the constant pH (acid) strategy and alkaline strategy are compared.

with the alkaline pH strategy were associated with a 65% (p<.01) augmentation in left ventricular performance (Fig. 2). Figure 7 demonstrates the immediate myocardial response in contractility resulting from increasing pH from 7.48 to 7.70.

Constant α (neutral) pH vs alkaline pH strategy – surface and perfusion hypothermia

In the constant α (neutral) pH group, arterial P_{CO_2} was kept at 35 to 40 mmHg throughout the entire temperature range (17 to 37°C). The meter and corrected

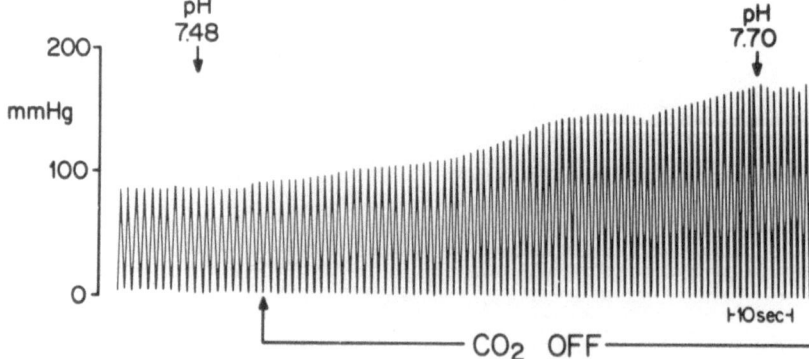

Fig. 7. Instantaneous changes in isovolumetric left ventricular pressure (balloon volume 25 ml) during perfusion hypothermia when P_{CO_2} was lowered to produce alkalosis. Note the marked increase in force of contraction resulting from pursuing the more alkaline strategy during perfusion hypothermia.

Table 1A. Blood gas analyses and hemodynamics during surface cooling.

Systemic temperature		37° C*	32° C*	27° C*	22° C*	17° C*
pH†	α (neutral)	7.40 ± 0.05	7.39 ± 0.04	7.41 ± 0.04	7.41 ± 0.04	7.39 ± 0.05
	alkaline	7.42 ± 0.05	7.58 ± 0.06+	7.69 ± 0.07+	7.80 ± 0.07+	7.85 ± 0.06+
P_{CO_2} (mmHg)	α (neutral)	40 ± 5	42 ± 5	45 ± 4	38 ± 4	39 ± 4
	alkaline	37 ± 5	20 ± 3+	14 ± 3+	11 ± 4+	10 ± 4+
Hct (%)	α (neutral)	33 ± 3	28 ± 3	24 ± 2	23 ± 2	22 ± 2
	alkaline	35 ± 3	26 ± 3	23 ± 2	21 ± 3	20 ± 3
Heart rate (min-l)	α (neutral)	155 ± 8	96 ± 7	60 ± 5	30 ± 7	–
	alkaline	160 ± 9	120 ± 8	86 ± 7+	44 ± 6	–
Syst. pressure (mmHg)	α (neutral)	102 ± 6	70 ± 5	60 ± 5	57 ± 5	–
	alkaline	107 ± 5	86 ± 4	76 ± 4+	70 ± 4+	–
Cardiac index	α (neutral)	102 ± 7	80 ± 7	63 ± 3	41 ± 3	–
(ml/kg/min)	alkaline	110 ± 8	105 ± 6+	96 ± 4+	64 ± 4+	–

Means ± SEM.
* Rectal temperature.
+ $p < 0.05$ from pH 7.4.
† pH meter reading (uncorrected).

Table 1B. Blood gas analyses, hemodynamics – pump cooling.

Systemic temperature		37° C*	32° C*	27° C*	22° C*	17° C*
pH	α (neutral)	7.41 ± 0.02	7.40 ± 0.02	7.39 ± 0.03	7.42 ± 0.04	7.41 ± 0.03
	alkaline	7.41 ± 0.02	7.55 ± 0.04+	7.66 ± 0.04+	7.75 ± 0.03+	7.82 ± 0.04+
P_{CO_2}	α (neutral)	35 ± 3	37 ± 4	39 ± 3	41 ± 3	41 ± 3
	alkaline	33 ± 3	22 ± 2+	16 ± 2+	13 ± 2+	9 ± 2+
Hct (%)	α (neutral)	35 ± 3	30 ± 3	28 ± 3	22 ± 3	21 ± 2
	alkaline	33 ± 2	30 ± 4	26 ± 4	23 ± 3	2 ± 3
Heart rate (min⁻¹)	α (neutral)	106 ± 8	115 ± 5	77 ± 6	41 ± 3	–
	alkaline	155 ± 9	108 ± 8	64 ± 4	39 ± 3	–
Pump flow † (ml/min)	α (neutral)	2025 ± 150	2625 ± 180	2375 ± 145	2000 ± 110	1800 ± 118
	alkaline	1850 ± 135	2000 ± 165	1975 ± 125	2200 ± 140	2550 ± 165+

Means ± SEM.
* Rectal temperature.
+ $p < 0.05$ from pH 7.4.
† 80 mmHg perfusion pressure.

Table 2A. Organ blood flow during surface cooling.

		37° C*	32° C*	27° C*	22° C*
LV flow†	α (neutral)	108 ± 8	70 ± 6	42 ± 3	29 ± 3
(cc/100 g/min)	alkaline	114 ± 9	77 ± 7	55 ± 5+	45 ± 4+
Kidney	α (neutral)	271 ± 41	234 ± 38	135 ± 32	62 ± 5
(cc/100 g/min)	alkaline	295 ± 52	282 ± 47	156 ± 35	83 ± 28
Cerebrum	α (neutral)	32 ± 3	24 ± 3	13 ± 2	10 ± 2
(cc/100 g/min)	alkaline	36 ± 4	34 ± 4	27 ± 3+	28 ± 3+
Brainstem	α (neutral)	40 ± 5	28 ± 4	18 ± 3	14 ± 2
(cc/100 g/min)	alkaline	39 ± 4	32 ± 3	29 ± 2+	27 ± +
Cerebellum	α (neutral)	42 ± 4	25 ± 4	20 ± 3	17 ± 2
(cc/100 g/min)	alkaline	40 ± 5	35 ± 5+	30 ± 3+	24 ± 3+

Means ± SEM.
* Rectal temperature.
+ $p < 0.05$ from pH 7.4.
† Subendocardium.

Table 2B. Body metabolism and organ blood flow – pump cooling.

		Pump cooling			Post rewarming
		37° C*	27° C*	22° C*	37° C*
Body O_2	α (neutral)	4.14 ± 0.22	1.90 ± 0.23	1.7 ± 0.30	5.25 ± 0.45
(cc/kg/min)	alkaline	4.20 ± 0.24	2.06 ± 0.33	1.64 ± 0.30	3.64 ± 0.34+
Body lactate	α (neutral)	14 ± 4	9 ± 2	2 ± 4	4 ± 3
(% extraction)	alkaline	8 ± 3	6 ± 4	18 ± 4	6 ± 2
Brain Blood flow	α (neutral)	28 ± 3	19 ± 2	14 ± 2	28 ± 4
(cc/100 g/min)	alkaline	31 ± 4	24 ± 3	20 ± 3	39 ± 5
Kidney Blood flow	α (neutral)	375 ± 35	205 ± 21	100 ± 18	278 ± 28
(cc/100 g/min)	alkaline	350 ± 28	210 ± 24	175 ± 16	310 ± 31

Means ± SEM.
* Rectal temperature.
+ $p < 0.05$ from pH 7.4.

pH values at different temperatures are shown in Fig. 3. In contrast P_{CO_2} is reduced progressively to $10 ± 4$ mmHg at 17° C in the pH adjusted group (Tables 1, 2).

Hemodynamics

With surface cooling, systolic blood pressure, heart rate, and cardiac index fell in all dogs as temperature was lowered (Fig. 8A, B). These hemodynamic indices were maintained at significantly higher levels in the alkaline pH group (Fig. 8A, B). Consequently there was better maintenance of total brain blood flow at 27°

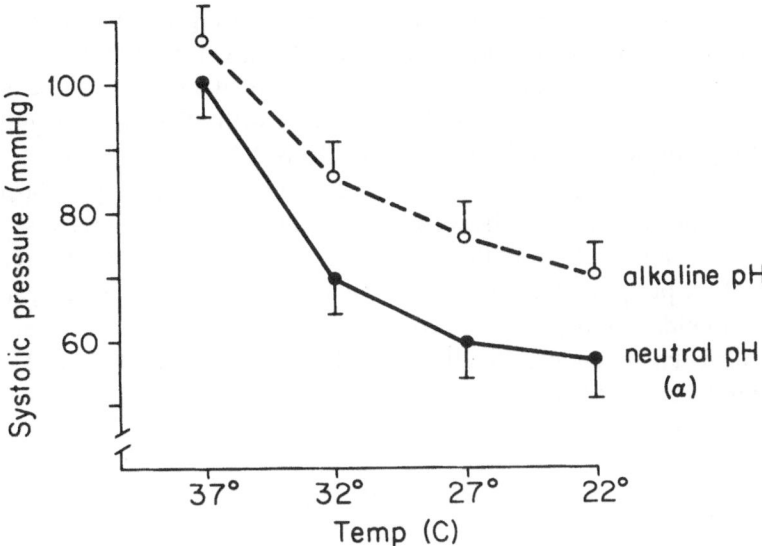

Fig. 8A. Arterial blood pressure during surface hypothermia.

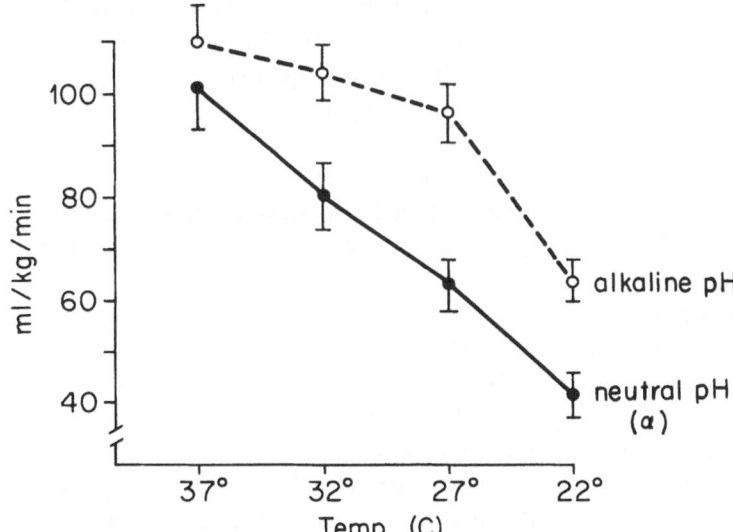

Fig. 8B. Cardiac index during surface hypothermia.

and 22° C with the alkaline pH strategy group despite the production of respiratory alkalosis by lowering P_{CO_2} to 14 and 11 mmHg, respectively (Fig. 9). The regional distribution of brain blood flow showed similar disparities between groups; at 22° C brain stem flow was reduced 56% in the constant α (neutral) pH group and only 34% in the alkaline strategy group while cerebral blood flow was reduced 60% vs 40% in each group, respectively (p<0.05). Renal blood flow was comparable in both groups during immersion hypothermia (Table 2a). Left ventricular blood flow decreased in both groups during cooling, with flow to the left subendocardial muscle maintained at 40% greater levels (p<0.05) in the alkaline pH group compared to when pH was kept at a meter reading of 7.4. For example, at 22° C LV flow was 45 cc/100 g/min with alkaline strategy, but only 29 cc/100 g/min with α (neutral) strategy (Table 2a).

With perfusion hypothermia, mean arterial pressure was kept at 80 mmHg by adjusting the flow in the extracorporeal circuit. Total peripheral vascular resistance was comparable in both groups with the exception of values recorded at 17° C, where peripheral resistance was higher with alkaline pH strategy (Table 3). Brain and kidney blood flow fell comparably in both groups, but total heart and left ventricular subendocardial flow was 50% higher in the alkaline pH group (91 vs 60 ml/100 gm/min) at 28° C.

Metabolism

With surface cooling, systemic oxygen utilization fell 80% as both cardiac index and blood pressure decreased with temperature in puppies whose pH was kept at a meter reading of 7.4, while following the constant α (neutral) pH strategy; progressive lactic acidosis (Fig. 10) developed in all puppies. In contrast, no puppy whose pH was made alkaline during surface cooling developed lactic acidosis while cardiac output and blood pressure were maintained at significantly higher levels (Fig. 10).

With perfusion hypothermia, systemic oxygen uptake was comparable in both pH groups and no systemic lactic acidosis developed as organ blood flow was maintained by the extracorporeal circuit which kept perfusion pressure at 80 mmHg (Table 2b).

With surface cooling, puppies kept in the constant α (neutral) pH strategy showed a progressive fall in left ventricular oxygen uptake per minute and left ventricular oxygen uptake/beat over the entire temperature range (Figs. 11A, B). The fall in cardiac oxygen uptake occurred coincident with a marked limitation of subendocardial flow and was associated with a progressive impairment of lactate metabolism; lactate production occurred at 22° C in the four puppy hearts which continued beating [7]. The two others developed ventricular fibrillations at 24 and 23° C, respectively. Ventricular fibrillation occurred at 22 ± 0.3° C in this group (Table 4). In contrast, hearts managed by the alkaline pH strategy showed

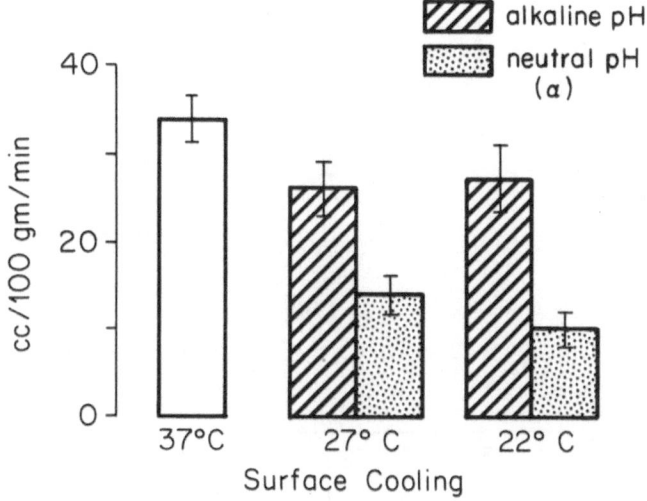

Fig. 9. Total brain blood flow during surface cooling. Note maintenance of cerebral perfusion in the alkaline strategy group.

Table 3. Acid-base-balance, systemic flow during rewarming.

Systemic temperature		Control before circ. arrest 17°	Rewarming (5 min. after reperfusion) 24°	32°	30 min. 37°	60 min. 37°
pH†	α (neutral)	7.39 ± 0.05	7.24 ± 0.04	7.32 ± 0.02	7.39 ± 0.02	7.42 ± 0.03
	alkaline	7.85 ± 0.06+	7.70 ± 0.04+	7.53 ± 0.03+	7.46 ± 0.02	7 .41 ± 0.02
Base excess	α (neutral)	−4 ± 1	−10 ± 2	−11 ± 3	−8 ± 2	−2 ± 0.5
	alkaline	−1 ± 0.5	−2 ± 0.5+	−1 ± 0.6+	−2 ± 1+	−2 ± 0.5
Pump flow++ ml/min	α (neutral)	700 ± 130	2,300 ± 350	3,100 ± 300	2,870 ± 60	3,300 ± 150
	alkaline	1,340 ± 160+	1,600 ± 14,0+	3,280 ± 200	3,420 ± 350	2,640 ± 210+

Means ± SEM.
* Rectal temperature.
+ p<0.05 from pH 7.4.
† pH meter reading (uncorrected).
++ 80 mmHg perfusion pressure.

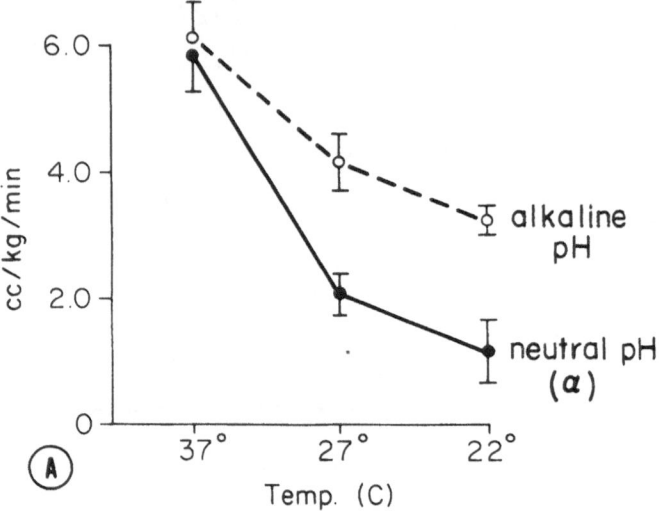

Fig. 10A. Systemic oxygen uptake during surface cooling.

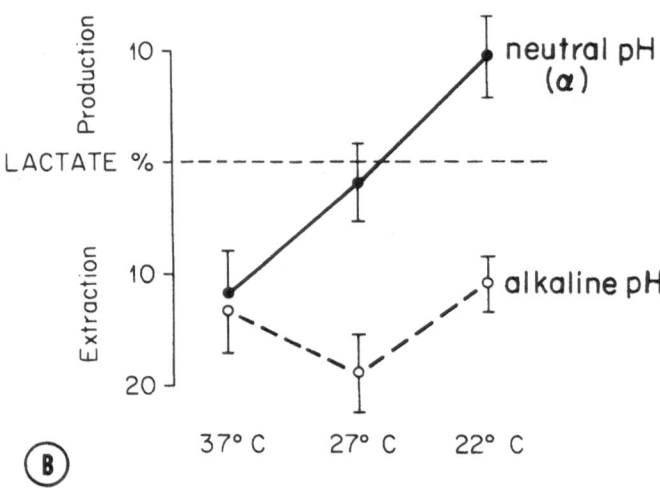

Fig. 10B. Systemic lactate metabolism during surface cooling.

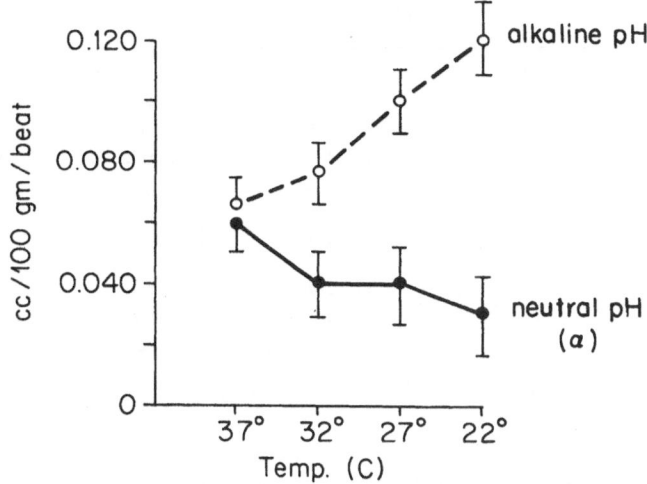

Fig. 11A. Left ventricular oxygen consumption per minute during surface cooling.

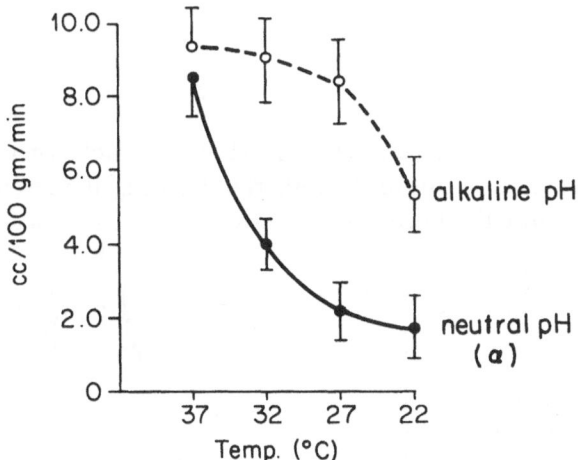

Fig. 11B. Left ventricular oxygen consumption per beat during surface cooling.

a progressive, but less pronounced fall in left ventricular oxygen uptake/minute (Fig. 11A). These hearts continued to consume lactate over the entire temperature range (Fig. 12). MVO_2/beat (Fig. 11B) increased progressively, reaching values approximately twice those at 37° C; regular cardiac rhythm was maintained in them until $17.7 \pm 5°$ C when ventricular fibrillation occurred.

With perfusion hypothermia, LVO_2 uptake/beat increased progressively but MVO_2/min fell as heart rate slowed while temperature was lowered. Left ventricular lactate consumption continued in all hearts, but was higher when pH was kept in the more alkaline range (5.9 vs 1.9 mg/100 g/min, $p < 0.05$ at 28° C).

Table 4.

	(n)	Cooling	Reperfusion	
		Fibrillation at °C+	No. of defibrillation	Sinus rhythm after (min)
pH α (neutral)	perfusion (8)	18.5 ± 0.4	0 ± 0	2.2 ± 0.4
	surface (6)	17.7 ± 0.5	0.5 ± 0.2	1.8 ± 0.5
pH alkaline	perfusion (8)	19.5 ± 0.6	3.0 ± 0.3*	10.2 ± 1.2*
	surface (6)	22.0 ± 0.3*	4.6 ± 1.1*	14.3 ± 1.6*

Means ± SEM.
* $p < 0.05$ from pH appr.
+ Rectal temperature.

Ventricular fibrillation occurred at comparable levels in both groups (18.5° C vs 17.7° C, Table 4) when perfusion pressure was maintained at 80 mmHg by the extracorporeal circuit.

Rewarming

Peripheral vascular resistance was lowest in both constant α (neutral) strategy pH groups (surface and perfusion hypothermia) during initiation of rewarming. Spontaneous ventricular fibrillation occurred coincident with aortic unclamping

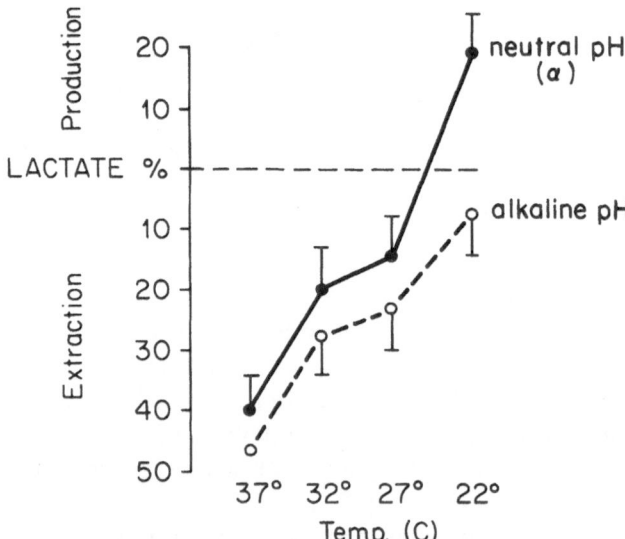

Fig. 12. Left ventricular lactate metabolism during surface cooling. Note: Myocardial lactate production of pH when the constant α (neutral) strategy is practiced and temperature is lowered below 28° C.

in all 14 hearts where the constant α (neutral) pH strategy was practiced and pH kept at 7.4 meter reading at 37°C during the period of reperfusion. Defibrillation was difficult; an average of 4.6 ± 1 and 3.0 ± 0.3 countershocks were required in the surface and perfusion hypothermia groups, respectively, and 14 ± 2 and 10 ± 1 minutes elapsed until regular sinus rhythm resumed (Table 4). In contrast, regular sinus rhythm resumed spontaneously in 13 of 14 hearts in the alkaline pH strategy group undergoing either surface or perfusion hypothermia. The only instance of ventricular fibrillation occurred in 1 dog undergoing surface cooling and required only one countershock for reversion.

Upon reperfusion, a washout lactate acidosis was seen in the constant α (neutral) pH strategy; pH was 7.24 during reperfusion while base excess was -10 ± 2 (p<0.05). In contrast, base excess during the initial phase of reperfusion was normal in the alkaline strategy groups (-2 ± 0.05) while pH was reduced progressively in these puppies as rewarming continued to 37°C (Table 3).

Left ventricular performance, evaluated by Starling function curves 30 minutes after reperfusion, was depressed significantly in both constant α (neutral) pH strategy groups. Stroke work index reached only 50% of control values at left atrial pressure of 25 mmHg (0.26 vs 1.27, p<0.05) after surface hypothermia and 75% (p<0.05) of control values in puppies undergoing perfusion hypothermia. Conversely, left ventricular performance was unchanged from control values in all hearts treated by the alkaline strategy during cooling and rewarming (Fig. 13) when either surface or perfusion hypothermia was used.

Discussion

This study was designed to simulate the conditions of cooling and rewarming before and after one hour of circulatory arrest with 'ideal' cardioplegic protection to determine the role of pH management on circulatory dynamics and eventual myocardial recovery. Our early studies of perfusion hypothermia demonstrated that following a constant pH (acid) strategy was less advantageous to total and left ventricular subendocardial flow, left ventricular metabolism and left ventricular performance than following an alkaline pH strategy. Subsequent studies of perfusion and surface hypothermia showed that following a constant α (neutral) pH strategy by keeping pH at 7.4 meter reading at 37°C during surface hypothermia produced the profound depression in cardiac output, cerebral and coronary blood flow, lactate acidosis and ultimate ventricular fibrillation reported by others [2–4]. This pH related inability of the heart to maintain organ blood flow was avoided if the constant α (neutral) strategy was practiced while cooling was achieved by perfusion hypothermia; the extracorporeal circuit ensured adequate perfusion vital organs. Repeated defibrillations were, however, necessary for cardiac resuscitation during rewarming and incomplete post-ischemic recovery of left ventricular function occurred whenever pH was kept in the constant α

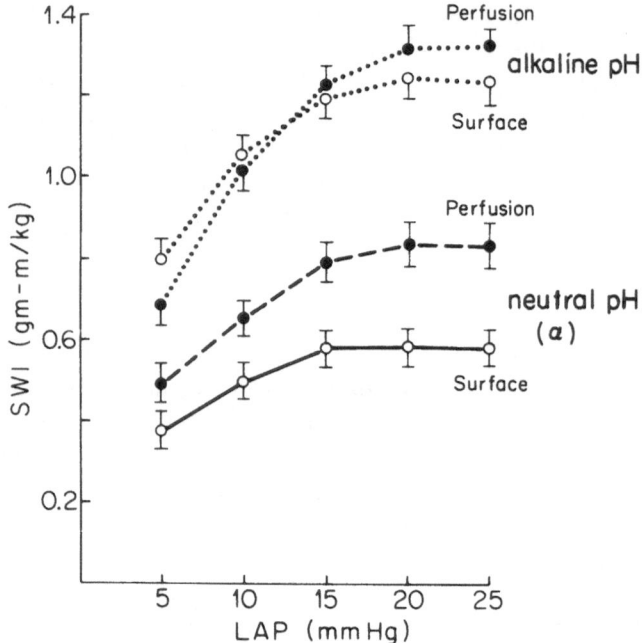

Fig. 13. Left ventricular performance after circulatory arrest. Normal postischemic left ventricular performance in alkaline strategy groups. Note: a) Normal post-ischemic left venticular performance in alkaline strategy groups. b) Significant depression when the constant α (neutral) is maintained during cooling and rewarming in the surface cooling group. c) Left depression when the constant α (neutral) strategy is used with perfusion hypothermia rather than surface cooling.

(neutral) strategy range during the cooling and rewarming phases. In contrast, applying a more alkaline strategy for pH management, in the highest range of values used by some cold blooded animals (ectotherms), allowed better maintenance of cardiac output and organ perfusion during cooling and prevented lactic acidosis and ventricular fibrillation. Regular cardiac rhythm resumed spontaneously during rewarming and myocardial performance recovered completely. These findings imply that failure of cardiac recovery after the clinical counterpart of this experiment may be avoided by appropriate adjustment of pH before and after circulatory arrest and cardioplegic protection.

Background

Most acid-base therapy is directed at keeping pH 7.4 at all temperatures because mammalian blood pH averages 7.40 at 37° C, and this pH is considered 'normal'. In 1932, Peters and Van Slyke [13] stated 'that for the maintenance of the organism in a state compatible with life, the reaction of the inner fluids must be slightly to the alkaline side of the neutral point and that much deviation from this physiologic reaction is disastrous'. Blood pH 7.40 at 37° C is, therefore, alkaline to the 6.8 neutral point of water at that temperature. Blood pH should increase with hypothermia if the concept of Peters and Van Slyke is valid, since blood pH at 7.4 would be considered 'acidotic' during hypothermia.

It is recognized from physical chemistry that the neutral point of water is temperature dependent and rises as temperature falls because of changes in its ionization constant (ΔpH/° C = 0.017) [14]. In 1948, Rosenthal reported similar physical chemical behaviour of in vitro mammalian blood samples held in gas tight syringes where a ΔpH/° C = 0.015 occurs when measurements in an enclosed eletrode system are made at various temperatures [8]. This factor is used in the clinical blood gas laboratories where blood samples taken from hypothermic patients are warmed at 37° C for analysis; results are reported either as measured (meter) or corrected values. For example, the pH of a blood sample from a patient at 17° C will be warmed to 37° C and then measured. The pH meter value would be 7.10, but the sample will be reported as a corrected value of 7.40.

The importance of reappraising our approach to pH management was recognized by Swan in 1974 [16]. In 1975, Rahn et al. [6] focused clinical attention on Howell's observation on ectotherms [5] by pointing out that an entire spectrum of vertebrates and invertebrates follow a thermal pattern whereby pH rises as temperature falls to maintain relative alkalinity [6]. These animals enter the realm of hypothermia as part of their natural conditions. The only exception to this rule seems to be the hibernating mammal who regularly keeps pH at 7.4 over a wide temperature range [15] (ΔpH/° C = 0.0). Rahn pointed out that the pH changes in ectotherms are due to the dominant effect of protein buffers, principally the imidazole of histadine. Rahn's review raised a justifiable questioning of proper pH regulation during hypothermia and stimulated a comparative physiologist colleague, Fred White [17], to call this issue to our attention at that time. Our early studies of perfusion hypothermia showed that cardiac function and metabolism were depressed and subendocardial perfusion reduced when a constant pH or acid strategy was followed in warm-blooded dogs whose temperature was lowered to 28° C. In contrast, raising pH by lowering P_{CO_2} of the extracorporeal circuit allowed the best myocardial metabolism performance at 28° C to occur at pH 7.72 [7]. This pH correction is at the very highest limits of the pH range reported in ectotherms (Fig. 1) and serves as a basis for the correction factor (ΔpH/° C = 0.33) used in current study, which may be termed the alkaline pH strategy.

Clinical practice

Most blood gas laboratories measure pH at 37° C, and clinical pH management during hypothermia follows 1 of 3 regimens. First, if there is awareness of the correction factor and adherence to keeping pH 7.4 at all temperatures, P_{CO_2} will be altered to achieve this pH level during hypothermia. For example, a 27° C, pH 7.55 blood sample analyzed at 37° C will have meter reading of 7.4, but be reported as pH 7.55 'corrected'. Under these circumstances, CO_2 would be added to achieve a 'corrected reading' of 7.4 at 27° C. This would be an acidotic pH for an ectotherm and a departure from the ideal suggested by Peters and Van Slyke. This is, however, the pattern practiced by hibernating animals (see Chapter 3) and perhaps is the most commonly used pH management in clinical practice. We tested this method only in our early pilot studies [7]. Such a strategy may be termed constant pH or acid strategy.

The constant pH or acid-base strategy has been chosen clinically because of the concept that 'normally a pH of 7.4 should prevail at all temperatures'. Certainly some justification for this approach can be derived from the data in warm-blooded hibernating mammals who follow this strategy in their natural habitat. There is, however, substantial evidence to suggest that such a strategy must be carefully re-evaluated when warm-blooded man, who does no hibernate, is placed into the unnatural world of hypothermia. It is well-recognized clinically that ventricular fibrillation develops when blood temperature is reduced below 28° C with surface cooling in the operating room setting, and cardiac arrest occurs in the non-clinical setting when warm blooded animals are exposed to severe cold (immersion hypothermia).

Second, if the constant α (neutral) pH strategy is considered to be ideal, and if the correction factor is either not applied or not reported, gas mixtures are adjusted by the anesthesiologists or perfusionist to keep pH 7.4 at 37° C. This method of pH management tests the hypothesis that pH management in warm-blooded man should follow ectothermic rules when we place him into the un-natural environment of hypothermia. We followed this regimen in the constant α (neutral) pH strategy group by keeping pH 7.4 at 37° C independent of body temperature. We recognized, of course, that true pH (temperature corrected) was higher and in the proper direction from a phylogenetic point of view (Fig. 1).

Third, pH may be varied to produce alkalosis by adjusting either P_{CO_2} [18, 19] or adding fixed base ($NaHCO_3$ or Tham) [20]. The concept of inducing respiratory alkalosis during hypothermia was introduced by Mohri several years ago [18] and used by us, based upon our previous study [7] to achieve an even greater degree of relative alkalosis in the current study. Regulation of P_{CO_2} to produce the desired pH during hypothermia carries the advantages of a) following phylogenetic tactics, b) ensuring rapid pH changes within the cell and consequent immediate buffering, and c) easier regulation during rewarming to avoid persistent meta-bolic alkalosis when pH 7.4 is desirable at warmer temperatures [20].

This method of pH management has no precedence in nature (i.e., hibernating animals or ectotherms). It must be realized however, that the surgical practice of a) entering euthermic (warm-blooded) humans into the world of ectotherms (cold-blooded animals), b) packing them in ice and placing them on car-diopulmonary bypass, c) anesthetizing them and paralyzing their respiratory drive while controlling their respiratory rate and depth, d) constraining their pH to levels defined arbitrarily as 'normal' (corrected or uncorrected), and e) shutting off their circulation for up to an hour also has no physiologic precedence in nature.

Our studies of surface cooling showed that systolic blood pressure and cardiac indices were maintained better when pH was manipulated to produce a level at the most alkaline range of ectotherms under similar conditions. In contrast, following the constant α (neutral) strategy resulted in a substantial fall in circulatory indices and metabolic evidence of inadequate cardiac output; systemic lactic acidosis developed in the same way as reported in clinical and experimental studies [2, 4, 12]. Conversely, systemic lactate metabolism remained normal when pH was adjusted to produce alkalosis during surface cooling.

We suspect the principal cause for better cardiac performance during surface hypothermia in alkaline pH strategy treated dogs was a more ideal biochemical environment for continued aerobic metabolism; left ventricular oxygen uptake/beat increased progressively (Fig. 11B) and no myocardial lactate production or ventricular fibrillation occurred. Conversely, a less ideal biochemical environment was evident during surface cooling when pH was kept in the constant α (neutral) strategy range (pH 7.4 meter reading at 37°C); subendocardial blood flow was maintained less well, myocardial lactate production occurred at 22°C and all dogs developed ventricular fibrillation at/or before 22°C was reached. Our findings are consistent with those of Rittenhouse who avoided ventricular fibrillation by producing moderate respiratory alkalosis during surface cooling to as low as 19°C [19]. We imposed more pronounced respiratory alkalosis and observed less fall in cardiac indices at low temperatures. Other causes for better cardiac performance include the inotropic effect of respiratory alkalosis [21] which may have added to the inotropic effect of hypothermia [22, 23] and accounted for the increased MVO_2/beat in dogs treated by the alkaline strategy. Based on the concept of relative alkalosis, pH 7.4 blood would be considered acidotic during hypothermia so that the constant pH strategy might be considered an acidotic strategy. The importance of avoiding intracellular acidosis during hypothermia is emphasized by studies of Poole-Wilson and Langer showing profound negative inotropic effect of respiratory acidosis at 24°C [24].

There has been proper reluctance to manage pH by reducing P_{CO_2} due to concern over cerebral hypoperfusion during hypocapnia at 37°C [25]. Our data show, however, that total and regional brain blood flow (cerebrum, brain stem, cerebellum) was maintained better (only 25% below control levels) in alkaline pH strategy treated dogs, despite lowering P_{CO_2} to 10 mmHg at 22°C (Fig. 9). Conversely, the marked cerebral hypoperfusion (75% below control values) produced by practicing the constant α (neutral) pH strategy was similar to that reported by others where higher P_{CO_2} levels were maintained [26–28]. We suspect that greater maintenance of systemic blood pressure and cardiac index allowed more adequate cerebral perfusion and that cerebral vasoregulation may have functioned better in the alkaline pH environment. The potential benefits of lowering P_{CO_2} and keeping pH higher during hypothermia are supported by the studies of Norwood *et al.* [29], showing that such pH manipulations ameliorate significantly the no-reflow lesions seen after anoxic cold brain perfusion. The profound cerebral hypoperfusion observed by following the constant α (neutral) pH strategy during surface cooling calls attention to the role of cerebral ischemia before circulatory arrest in causing post-operative neurologic problems. Cerebral blood flow was comparable to both constant α (neutral) and alkaline strategies in the perfusion hypothermia groups, as the deleterious hemodynamic effects were avoided by ensuring organ blood flow by taking over the function of the heart in those studies where all cooling was accomplished by the extracorporeal circuit. Unfortunately, we did not test whether perfusion hypothermia would maintain cerebral blood flow during the pH constant or acid strategy. These data demonstrating the satisfactory maintenance of organ blood flow when perfusion hypothermia is used to keep blood pressure high suggest that strict adherence to the alkaline strategy may be less critical during perfusion hypothermia, unless a period of circulatory arrest is contemplated.

All dogs were given the same myocardial protection (multidose cold blood cardioplegia) during the one hour period of circulatory arrest because this treatment prevents damage for up to two hours of aortic clamping in adult dogs. Multidose cardioplegia may have been unnecessary since noncoronary collateral washout cannot occur during circulatory arrest. Avoidance of any myocardial damage during aortic clamping was essential in our study to assess the effects of the events before and after circulatory arrest and cardioplegia. The completeness of recovery in all hearts subjected to the alkaline pH strategy suggests that myocardial protection was excellent. Conversely, failure to recover completely after the constant α (neutral) pH strategy indicates that failure to follow a more alkaline pH strategy during hypothermia was responsible for the myocardial changes.

Systemic lactate acidosis developed in all dogs during circulatory arrest so that pH was low during the initial phase of rewarming despite a reversal of the pattern of pH regulation. Systemic vascular resistance was 30% ($p < 0.05$) lower when cardiopulmonary bypass was restarted in the constant α (neutral) pH group, presumably because more acid metabolites accumulated in these dogs; base excess recovered more slowly in them. Reperfusion systemic acidosis was less severe when the constant α (neutral) strategy was practiced during perfusion hypothermia, in preference to surface cooling. Presumably, better maintenance of organ blood flow during cooling reduced the extent of acidosis before circulatory arrest. An additional potential benefit of the alkaline strategy may be that the extra buffering effect of a more alkaline pH at the onset of circulatory arrest may have delayed the buildup of acid metabolites which occurs when extracorporeal circulation is discontinued. This effect may be similar to that which occurs when hyperventilation is practiced before breath holding in an effort to increase the tolerance to a given period of anoxia.

Acid-base balance was, of course, restored to normal when post-ischemic ventricular performance was tested in all animals. Usually, regular sinus rhythm resumes spontaneously in dogs protected by multidose cold blood cardioplegia and this occurred in 13 of 14 hearts when the alkaline pH strategy was practiced. Conversely, each dog treated by the constant α (neutral) strategy developed ventricular fibrillation during reperfusion, and repeated defibrillations were necessary before regular rhythm was established (averaging 10–14 minutes). The persistence of ventricular fibrillation during the early phase of rewarming may have impaired subendocardial perfusion and contributed to the myocardial depression seen 30 minutes later.

Left ventricular performance returned to pre-ischemic level in all dogs treated by the alkaline pH strategy. Conversely, 50% depression of post-ischemic performance occurred in hearts receiving the same cardioplegic protection where the constant α (neutral) pH strategy during surface cooling was imposed and 25% depression occurred when perfusion hypothermia was used with this strategy.

All hearts could support the circulation spontaneously but a higher left atrial pressure was required to keep the same level of stroke work index. Histologic studies were not obtained to determine if these changes were irreversible. We interpret the complete recovery of myocardial performance in the alkaline pH strategy group to indicate that failure to recover completely in the others was due to inappropriate pH management before and after circulatory arrest and aortic clamping, rather than a limitation of cardioplegic protection per se. The better recovery seen in the constant α (neutral) strategy perfusion hypothermia group likely was due to less severe myocardial damage prior to circulatory arrest since the heart was cooled in the beating empty state while its perfusion was assured by maintenance of adequate blood pressure in the extracorporeal circuit.

The slope for ideal pH for human hearts during hypothermia is unknown, but our findings imply that higher level mammalian hearts function better in the more alkalotic range when we enter them into realm of hypothermia. Our data in the constant α (neutral) pH strategy group, where CO_2 content was held relatively constant as in poikilotherms showed that a strict poikilothermic strategy is less effective than a more alkalotic strategy. Fortunately, the availability of extracorporeal circulation to ensure vital organ perfusion and avoid ventricular fibrillation in the perfusion hypothermia studies allowed us to circumvent the myocardial depression caused by following strict constant α (neutral) pH strategy in the euthermic animal placed in the unnatural environment of hypothermia. We did not test the constant pH (acid) strategy during surface hypothermia or with circulatory arrest, but extrapolation of our data on the results of this strategy with perfusion hypothermia would infer that such pH management would be even less ideal than keeping pH following the constant α (neutral) pH strategy. Further study of this problem is indicated.

Our findings relate directly to cardiac procedures where surface cooling and perfusion hypothermia are practiced and suggest that reappraisal of pH management during hypothermia should be undertaken. Such information may have additional application of other areas of hypothermic organ preservation. Studies by *Halasz* show that cold preservation of rabbit and canine kidneys at pH in the alkaline range of 7.4 result in better recovery of function and less lysozymal enzyme release [30].

We conclude from this study that pH 7.4 may not be either 'normal' or 'ideal' during hypothermia. Constraining pH 7.4, corrected or uncorrected, during hypothermia causes a degree of myocardial damage and limitation of myocardial protection which is avoidable by pH adjustment during cooling and rewarming to a position in the most alkaline range seen in ectotherms. These findings may have major implications in the routine management of hypothermia during all cardiac operations.

References

1. Barratt-Boyes BG, Simpson M, Neutze JM: Intracardiac surgery in neonates and infants using deep hypothermia with surface cooling and limited cardiopulmonary bypass. Circulation 43, 44: Suppl 1: 125, 1971.
2. Johnston AE, Radde IC, Steward DJ, Taylor J: Acid-base and electrolyte changes in infants undergoing profound hypothermia for surgical correction of congenital heart defects. Can Anaesth Soc J 21: 23, 1974.
3. Steward DJ, Sloan IA, Johnston AE: Anaesthetic management of infants undergoing profound hypothermia for surgical correction of congenital heart defects. Canad Anaesth Soc J 21: 15, 1974.
4. Shida H, Morimoto M, Inokawa K, Tsugane J, Ikeda Y: Simple deep hypothermia for open-heart surgery. J Cardiovasc Surg 20: 135, 1979.
5. Howell BJ, Baumgardner FW, Bondi K, Rahn H: Acid-base balance in cold-blooded vertebrates as a function of body temperature. Am J Physiol 218: 600, 1970.
6. Rahn H, Reeves RB, Howell BJ: Hydrogen ion regulation, temperature, and evolution. Am Rev Respir Dis 112: 165, 1975.
7. McConnell DH, White F, Nelson RL, Goldstein SM, Maloney JV Jr, DeLand EC, Buckberg GD: Importance of alkalosis in maintenance of 'ideal' blood pH during hypothermia. Surg Forum 26: 263, 1975.
8. Rosenthal TB: The effects of temperature on the pH of blood and plasma in vitro. J Biol Chem 173: 25, 1948.
9. Behar MG, Severinghaus JW: Calibration and a correction of blood O_2 content measured by P_{O_2} after CO saturation. J Appl Physiol 29: 413, 1970.
10. Buckberg GD, Fixler DE, Archie JP, Hoffman JIE: Experimental subendocardial ischemia in dogs with normal coronary arteries. Circ Res 30: 67, 1972.
11. Follette DM, Mulder DG, Maloney JV Jr, Buckberg GD: Advantages of blood cardioplegia over continuous coronary perfusion and intermittent ischemia. An experimental and clinical study. J Thorac Cardiovasc Surg 76: 604, 1978.
12. Bigelow WG, Lindsay WK, Greenwood WF: Hypothermia: its possible role in cardiac surgery. An investigation of factors governing survival in dogs at low body temperatures. Ann Surg 132: 849, 1950.
13. Peters JP, Van Slyke DD: Quantitative Clinical Chemistry. The Williams & Wilkins Company, Baltimore, 1932: 868.

14. Austin JH, Cullen GE: Hydrogen ion concentration of the blood in health and disease. Medicine 4: 275, 1925.
15. Goodrich CA: Acid-base balance in ectothermic and hibernating marmots. Am J Physiol 224: 1185, 1973.
16. Swan H: Thermoregulation and Bioenergetics – Patterns for Vertebrate Survival. American Elsevier Publishing Co., New York, 1974.
17. White FN: Temperature and the Galapagos marine iguana. Insights into reptilian thermoregulation. Comp Biochem Physiol 45A: 503, 1973.
18. Mohri H, Dillard DH, Crawford EW, Martin WE, Merendino KA: Method of surface-induced deep hypothermia for open-heart surgery in infants. J Thorac Cardiovasc Surg 58: 262, 1969.
19. Rittenhouse EA, Ito CS, Mohri H, Merendino KA: Circulatory dynamics during surface-induced deep hypothermia and after cardiac arrest for one hour. J Thorac Cardiovasc Surg 61: 359, 1971.
20. Ellis RJ, Hoover E, Gay WA, Ebert PA: Metabolic alterations with profound hypothermia. Arch Surg 109: 659, 1974.
21. Streisand RL, Gourin A, Stuckey JH: Respiratory and metabolic alkalosis and myocardial contractility. J Thorac Cardiovasc Surg 62: 431, 1971.
22. Buckberg GD, Brazier JR, Nelson RL, Goldstein SM, McConnell DH, Cooper N: Studies of the effects of hypothermia on regional myocardial blood flow and metabolism during cardiopulmonary bypass. I. The adequately perfused beating, fibrillating and arrested heart. J Thorac Cardiovasc Surg 73: 87, 1977.
23. Monroe RG, Strange RH, LaFarge CG, Levy J: Ventricular performance, pressurevolume relationship, and O_2 consumption during hypothermia. Am J Physiol 206: 67, 1964.
24. Poole-Wilson PA, Langer GA: Effect of pH on ionic exchange and function in rate and rabbit myocardium. Am J Physiol 229: 570, 1975.
25. Reivich M: Arterial P_{CO_2} and cerebral hemodynamics. Am J Physiol 206: 25, 1964.
26. Kawashima Y, Okada K, Kosugi I, In-nami H, Yamaguchi Y, Fujihara T, Yamamura H: Changes in distribution of cardiac output by surface-induced deep hypothermia in dogs. J Appl Physiol 40: 876, 1976.
27. Su JY, Amory DW, Sands MP, Mohri H: Effects of ether anesthesia and surface induced hypothermia on regional blood flow. Am Heart J 97: 53, 1979.
28. Rudy LW, Boucher JK, Edmunds LH: The effect of deep hypothermia and circulatory arrest on the distribution of system blood flow in rhesus monkeys. J Thorac Cardiovasc Surg 64: 706, 1972.
29. Norwood WI, Norwood DR, Castaneda AR: Cerebral anoxia. Effect of deep hypothermia and pH. Surgery 86: 203, 1979.
30. Halasz NA, Collins GM, White FN: The right pH for preservation? Organ Preservation, Vol III, D Pegg, ed., London, 1979, Churchill Livingstone, p. 259.

Subject index